Neurological Examination
Second Edition

pocket tutor

Neurological Examination
Second Edition

pocket tutor

John A Goodfellow BSc (Hons)
BM BCh MRCP (UK) PhD
Clinical Lecturer in Neurology
University of Glasgow
Glasgow, UK

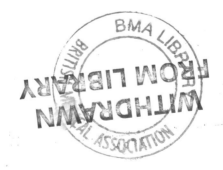

JP
medical
publishers

© 2018 JP Medical Ltd.

First edition 2012

Published by JP Medical Ltd, 83 Victoria Street, London, SW1H 0HW, UK

Tel: +44 (0)20 3170 8910   Fax: +44 (0)20 3008 6180

Email: info@jpmedpub.com   Web: www.jpmedpub.com

ISBN: 978-1-909836-70-9

British Library Cataloguing in Publication Data
A catalogue record for this book is available from the British Library

Library of Congress Cataloging in Publication Data
A catalog record for this book is available from the Library of Congress

Publisher:	Richard Furn
Development Editor:	Thomas Banister-Fletcher
Editorial Assistant:	Adam Rajah
Design:	Designers Collective Ltd

Foreword

An increasing trend towards sub-specialisation in later practice makes it more essential than ever that all doctors grasp the fundamentals of performing a neurological examination as early as possible. The first edition of *Pocket Tutor Neurological Examination* proved a popular and dependable guide for both students and junior doctors. This new edition has many new examination photographs, full-colour figures and diagrams, refined descriptions of examination technique and an expanded section on developments in the management of acute stroke.

These improvements add to a practical and highly accessible book that will demystify neurological assessment.

Martin R Turner
Consultant Neurologist
John Radcliffe Hospital, Oxford
Richard & Joan Doll Clinical Tutorial Fellow
Green Templeton College
University of Oxford, UK

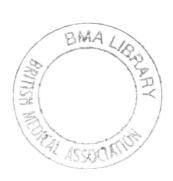

Preface

Pocket Tutor Neurological Examination presents the neurological examination in a way that is both accessible and clinically useful. Medical students should find it has enough detail to help them pass their final examinations with confidence and, equally, junior doctors will find enough information to feel confident when making a general assessment in routine clinical practice.

This second edition of *Pocket Tutor Neurological Examination* has been updated and revised in response to feedback on the first edition. The diagrams are now full colour and there are more photographs showing examination technique and signs. Several chapters have been expanded, with the chapter on examining the stroke patient now covering neurosurgical procedures and thrombectomy in addition to thrombolysis.

With its compact size, system summaries highlighting the essentials at the end of each chapter and additional practical tips, *Pocket Tutor Neurological Examination* provides students and junior doctors with a concise summary of the fundamentals and a comprehensive overview of the subject.

I hope you enjoy this second edition.

John Goodfellow
January 2018

Contents

Acknowledgements

From the author
Many thanks to Rosalyn for her support and encouragement through this project. Thank you to all my colleagues who teach me something new about neurology each day.

From the publisher
The photo used in Figure 3.7 was originally published in *Pocket Tutor Surface Anatomy* (© 2012 JP Medical Ltd) and is reproduced courtesy of Sam Scott-Hunter, London, UK.

Clinical skills in neurology

1.1 The consultation

The majority of clinical neurology is practised in the outpatient setting, usually by consultants or registrars. However, neurological emergencies and chronic neurological conditions are common enough that every junior doctor needs to be skilled in their assessment and key areas of management.

The key clinical skill in neurology is history taking. This stage will almost always be the most informative, and time well spent here will make the rest of the consultation more meaningful. The history and other areas of the consultation enable the lesion to be localised and likely pathological processes identified.

Rather than the history, the physical examination is the part that most inexperienced juniors are nervous about and likely to spend most time on. The value of the examination is in confirming abnormalities suspected from the history and in detecting dysfunction not reported by the patient, thereby further assisting in localising the lesion. If the history is taken properly, there should be no surprises!

Investigations should be considered as an extension of the physical examination, that is, to confirm or refute specific findings from the history or examination. Many patients who consult a neurologist expect a brain scan, but this is not always in their interest; most patients can be reassured by nothing more than a thorough history and examination.

1.2 The neurological history

This is the central aspect of the neurology consultation. The aims are:

1. understand the patient in their individual context
2. detect abnormal symptoms that suggest a lesion
3. localise the lesion through knowledge of neuroanatomy

4. identify potential pathogenic processes, largely though establishing the time course and progression of symptoms and the remainder of the medical history

When taking the neurological history, always ask yourself the question 'Which part of the nervous system would have to be damaged to produce these symptoms?'

Meeting the patient

When first meeting the patient:
- ask their name, age, handedness and employment history
- establish rapport

> ### Clinical insight
>
> A good way to build rapport with the patient is to start the consultation by asking what their job is, who they live with and what they would like to get out of the consultation. Introduce yourself to whoever is attending with the patient; they are probably the most significant person in their life and will be able to offer some useful input.

Presenting complaint

To determine more about the presenting complaint, ask an open question to identify the patient's main concern, such as 'What is the main problem?' If there are multiple problems, approach them separately and in turn.

History of presenting complaint

For each problem establish:
- the time of onset: 'When were you last well in this regard?'
- progression: 'How has it changed since it started?'
- relation to other symptoms: 'Which came first? Then what?'
- time course
- aggravating and relieving factors

Time course

Establishing the time course of symptoms is crucial but easily passed over. Determine as exactly as possible the day, week or month of symptom onset, the order of onset of symptoms and their progression.

The differential diagnosis of neurological conditions is greatly influenced by whether the symptoms are acute, sub-acute or chronic.

Neurological systems review

Specifically ask the patient about each of the following, and then explore any findings as above:

- loss of consciousness
- abnormal movements
- headaches
- weakness
- sensory symptoms
- balance problems
- visual problems
- seizures
- speech problems
- memory or planning problems
- skin problems
- infections

Past medical history

When taking the past medical history:

- establish all previous medical and surgical problems
- include any childhood illnesses
- clarify dates and precise meanings of any medical terms the patient uses

Social history

This places the patient in their social context and allows you to assess the full impact of the illness on them. When indicated, focus on the following aspects:

> **Clinical insight**
>
> Always clarify what a patient means when they use medical jargon or diagnostic terms. They may mean something completely different from the established meaning!

- employment history ('What age were you when you left school?', 'What was your first job?', 'What was your next?', etc.), including occupational exposure to chemicals and other potential hazards
- travel history
- unusual diet
- smoking and alcohol history

- recreational drug use
- human immunodeficiency virus and other blood-borne virus risk factors
- where the patient lives and with whom
- levels of stress at home and at work

Family history

To determine the family history:
- draw out a family tree
- include all causes of death, neurological illness and other major illnesses

Clinical insight

It is often easier to ask about the 'family dynamics', the psychiatric history and what the patient thinks is wrong with them and why at the first consultation. This is a thorough approach to history-taking, and is usually perceived as such by the patient. It also makes it easier to return to discussing these topics if they are subsequently thought to be important contributors to the presenting problem (e.g. dissociative seizures).

Drug history

A full drug history should be taken. The current or past use of antidopaminergic drugs should be documented in patients with movement disorders.

Systems review

Thorough questioning about other systems should be carried out:

- include cardiac, renal, respiratory, gastrointestinal, psychiatric and ophthalmological symptoms as standard
- ask yourself whether the neurological disease is contributing to the systemic symptoms, whether disease of another system is contributing to neurological symptoms or whether there is an underlying multisystem disease

1.3 The neurological examination

At the end of the history there should be a number of neurological symptoms detected and a range of differential diagnoses to account for them. The subsequent examination will be either a brief screening examination or a more thorough assessment.

A succinct screening exam is appropriate when the likelihood of signs is low (e.g. in patients with suspected simple migraine), whereas a detailed assessment is appropriate if the differentials include disorders likely to have physical signs, for instance, in patients with suspected cervical myelopathy.

Patients sometimes find the neurological examination to be a strange experience, with a doctor asking them to obey odd instructions that seem completely unrelated to their reasons for seeking medical attention ('I've been having double vision so why is the doctor asking me to stand on my feet and close my eyes?'). Explain at the outset that the purpose of the tests is not only to assess the problem they have but also to assess the function of the rest of their brain and the nerves and muscles in the rest of their body.

The remaining chapters describe the various parts of the examination. With experience, it becomes easier to decide how detailed an exam needs to be and how to focus the exam according to the differentials. For example, in acute stroke, a brief but targeted screening examination (see Chapter 9) allows classification of the stroke syndrome, which is important for immediate management decisions, but does not delay treatment by searching for minor neurological signs. In contrast, patients with Guillain–Barré syndrome need detailed assessment of all peripheral nerves to enable close monitoring of progression.

1.4 Case summary and synthesis

The neurological case is often lengthy and detailed in terms of the complete history and examination findings. It is helpful to routinely summarise the relevant positive and negative findings when writing in the case notes. This step helps to clarify the case and synthesise the various elements. It should come after the examination findings and consist of just a paragraph or two of the findings. This should be followed by an opinion on the differential diagnosis and a plan for further investigation, treatment and other management.

1.5 Describing and referring cases

Summarising a patient's neurological problems can be daunting because the history and examination findings are often complex. The key is having thought through the case and being clear what the relevant positive and negative findings are. It is helpful to start the case presentation or referral with a brief summary that highlights the working diagnosis and/or management plan. For example, if referring a patient with suspected cauda equina to a neurosurgeon, it would be helpful to begin with:

'This 35-year-old right-handed man with new-onset lower back pain presents with saddle anaesthesia, faecal and urinary incontinence, absent ankle reflexes and weakness in ankle plantar flexion, consistent with cauda equina syndrome.'

In an examination situation the examiners may simply allow you, the candidate, to proceed to describe the usual history and examination findings. However, since you have already clearly identified and summarised these with this sentence, the impressed examiner may in fact skip this altogether and ask about investigation and management, thereby allowing more advanced discussion.

When referring patients to neurologists, for example over the phone, it is helpful to begin with a brief summary or background such as the one quoted above. This shows

> **Clinical insight**
>
> **How to summarise a case**
>
> **Suspected multiple sclerosis:** example case summary
>
> A 27-year-old, female, right-handed supermarket worker presents with a 2-week history of slowly progressive paraesthesias in both legs. Her past medical history includes an episode of transient right visual loss 2 years ago, and a 2-week episode of acute ataxia and vertigo 6 months ago. Examination reveals a sensory loss of pin prick to her skin to the region of the T10 dermatome, clonus in both ankles and brisk knee reflexes. There is no family history of multiple sclerosis or other neurological disease.
>
> **Opinion:** multiple sclerosis seems a likely diagnosis. Other causes of multifocal CNS disease need to be excluded.
>
> **Plan:** MRI brain and spinal cord; lumbar puncture for cell count, protein and glucose, and oligoclonal bands; consider visual-evoked potentials if the above is not diagnostic.

that the patient has been carefully assessed and indicates the purpose of the referral.

1.6 The junior doctor's neurology toolkit

Figure 1.1 shows the author's own 'junior doctor's neurology toolkit'. This is a collection of tools for routine neurological assessment on general hospital wards.
It includes:

- an ophthalmoscope for fundoscopy
- tropicamide (a pupil dilator): can be obtained from an ophthalmology ward or emergency department and is used to allow better examination of the retina
- tuning forks for vibration sense testing (assessing the dorsal columns)
- pins for pin-prick testing (assessing the lateral columns)
- a few small objects (e.g. key, battery) are good for assessing stereognosis
- tongue depressors and throat swabs are helpful when the gag reflex needs to be formally tested

It is also useful to carry a Snellen pocket chart for testing acuity and to use Ishihara plates, e.g. on a smartphone, when indicated. A variety of tools are available for bedside screening of cognition. For example, the Queen Square Screening Test for Cognitive Deficits is a small book available directly from the

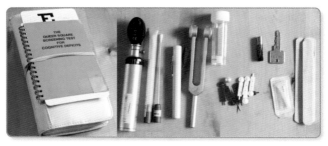

Figure 1.1 The junior doctor's neurology toolkit.

National Hospital for Neurology and Neurosurgery in London. The Addenbrooke's cognitive examination is a shorter alternative, freely available online.

1.7 Ethicolegal considerations

The diagnosis of a neurological condition often carries significant and lifelong morbidity and social restrictions as well as having implications for driving and obtaining life or travel insurance. Patients should be referred to someone with experience in dealing with these issues to make them aware of the implications of their diagnosis and answer any queries they have.

Driving restrictions

There are driving restrictions for those diagnosed with certain neurological disorders, and such a patient should be referred to the relevant public authority [e.g. the Driver and Vehicle Licensing Agency (DVLA) in the UK] for up-to-date details on driving restrictions. Some patients will be eligible for disability welfare support [e.g. Disability Living Allowance (DLA) in the UK].

Expectations of imaging

Many patients expect or want some form of neuroimaging for reassurance. Although it is now relatively straightforward to obtain this for almost any neurological symptom, it is important to discuss a number of issues with patients. CT scanning involves radiation exposure and is not, strictly speaking, a harmless investigation.

MRI avoids this but often identifies incidental abnormalities that are unrelated to the presenting problem and of uncertain significance. This occurs in around 10% of scans and is a major consideration in the design and implementation of neuroimaging research studies that utilise 'normal' controls. As well as increasing anxiety in patients, there may also be health and travel insurance implications.

Gait and general inspection

The initial general inspection and observation of gait should be done in all patients. There are far too many neurological syndromes to know, let alone summarise here. However, a few are sufficiently common or important that the generalist should be aware of them. Abnormalities of posture and movement should be precisely described in order to direct further investigation. The nomenclature can be confusing, but a few moments of reflection on the groups of muscles involved, the nature of the movement and a few other features allows a straightforward classification.

2.1 Anatomy and physiology review

Posture can be thought of as a steady state requiring ongoing co-ordination of sensory input and motor commands. Abnormal postures can reflect abnormal input, integration or motor output. Abnormal movements are the result of dysfunction somewhere within this complex neural system.

Sensory input

The dorsal column–medial lemniscus pathway carries proprioceptive input from the joints and muscles in the periphery to the dorsal column of the spinal cord. It ascends ipsilaterally to the level of the medulla, where the primary sensory neurons synapse on secondary neurons in the cuneate and gracile nuclei (**Figure 2.1**) (see Figure 4.4). These then decussate (the internal arcuate fibres) and ascend as the medial lemniscus to synapse on neurons in the ventral posteromedial and ventral posterolateral nuclei in the thalamus. From here there are diffuse projections, most importantly via the internal capsule to the primary sensory cortex (the postcentral gyrus).

The vestibular system provides sensory information about body position and balance. The vestibular nuclei are anatomically and functionally closely linked with the cerebellar nuclei and are discussed in more detail in Chapter 6.

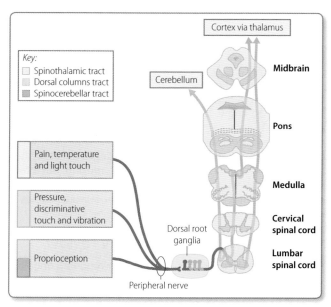

Figure 2.1 Major sensory pathways. The dorsal columns mainly carry light touch, vibration sense and proprioception. The spinothalamic or 'lateral columns' carry mainly pain, temperature and light touch.

Pyramidal system

The pyramidal system describes a major component of the control of movement whose main outflow tract is via the 'pyramids' in the brainstem. This largely comprises the corticospinal tract.

The corticospinal tract begins with the pyramidal cells of layer V of the primary motor cortex (these are called pyramidal because of their shape, not because they are part of the pyramidal system). Their axons pass through the internal capsule and form the pyramidal tract.

> ### Guiding principle
>
> **Dorsal column–medial lemniscus pathway**: proprioceptive fibres → ipsilateral dorsal column → cuneate and gracile nuclei in the medulla → cross as the internal arcuate fibres → ascend in the medial lemniscus → ventral posteromedial and ventral posterolateral nuclei in the thalamus → primary sensory cortex.

90% of pyramidal tract fibres cross sides (decussate) in the medulla; the remainder stay ipsilateral (**Figure 2.2**).

These fibres travel down to the α-motor neurons in the anterior horn of the spinal cord (or the motor neuron in the cranial nerve nuclei), which they directly synapse onto (mostly excitatory) or indirectly synapse through a complex network of interneurons (mostly inhibitory).

> ### Guiding principle
>
> **Pyramidal system**: layer V pyramidal cells in the motor cortex → internal capsule → cross at the pyramidal decussation in the medulla → synapse on α-motor neurons and interneurons in the anterior horn of the spinal cord.

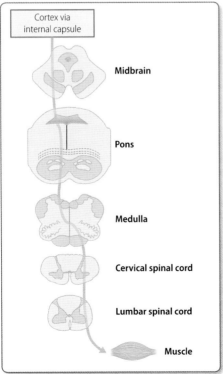

Figure 2.2 The pyramidal system. The descending corticospinal tract is the main pathway for voluntary control of movement.

Cortex via internal capsule

Midbrain

Pons

Medulla

Cervical spinal cord

Lumbar spinal cord

Muscle

This system controls much of voluntary movement and is also a major pathway for the extrapyramidal control of movements.

Basal ganglia/extrapyramidal system

The basal ganglia includes the:

- striatum
- globus pallidus
- substantia nigra
- subthalamic nucleus

Their inputs, internal connections and output pathways are very complex (**Figure 2.3**). A detailed knowledge is not required for clinical practice except in the rare cases of small unilateral lesions and for functional neurosurgery for movement disorders. The clinical syndromes that are caused by basal ganglia dysfunction are classified on clinical grounds rather than on anatomical localisation of the lesions.

The basal ganglia affect cognition, emotion and, in particular, movement. They are involved in selecting individual actions and motor plans. They are therefore at the centre of motor function, between planning and execution.

Clinical insight

Hemiballismus is an involuntary flinging movement of a limb, most commonly caused by a stroke. It is usually caused by a lesion in the contralateral subthalamic nucleus. The lesion reduces the excitatory input to the globus pallidus from the subthalamic nucleus. This in turn disinhibits the thalamus, which thereby increases its excitatory output to the cortex, resulting in the hyperkinetic movements. It is a loss of descending inhibition.

Cerebellum

There are more neurons in the cerebellum than in the rest of the brain. The cerebellum is located in the posterior fossa and forms the roof of the fourth ventricle. It is covered in more detail in Chapter 6. Briefly, its chief function is the execution and control of fine movements, ensuring proper timing and accuracy in particular. It is a major site for the control of learned or automatic

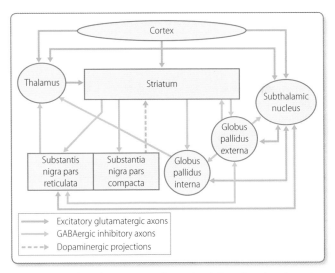

Figure 2.3 Basal ganglia connections. Dopaminergic input from the substantia nigra and input from the motor cortex are modulated as they pass through the pallidum and back into the thalamus and cortex. There are separate, parallel, direct and indirect loops through the GPi and GPe/subthalamic nuclei back to the thalamus and cortex. GPe, globus pallidus external; GPi, globus pallidus internal; SNr, substantia nigra pars reticulata; SNc, substantia nigra pars compacta.

movements. It can be thought of as a massive switchboard, connecting incoming cortical and basal ganglia movement plans with the cerebellar output nuclei, which in turn project back to the spinal cord, vestibular nuclei and cerebral cortex.

It comprises two cerebellar hemispheres connected by the vermis. The flocullonodular lobe is tucked in at the base. There is somatotopic organisation with the head represented on the anterior lobe, the upper limbs and upper trunk more posteriorly and the lower limbs and lower trunk more posteriorly still. The midline of the body is represented on the vermis and the distal limbs laterally.

2.2 Clinical features and pathophysiology

General inspection

Syndromes

These include:

- Parkinson's disease
- Bell's palsy (idiopathic inflammation of the facial nerve)
- acromegaly
- myasthenia gravis
- Sturge–Weber syndrome (encephalotrigeminal angioma-tosis)
- Huntington's disease
- ataxia telangiectasia
- Charcot–Marie–Tooth disease (hereditary motor and sensory neuropathy (HMSN))
- dermatomyositis
- myotonic dystrophy
- neurofibromatosis
- tuberous sclerosis
- Wilson's disease (hepatolenticular degeneration)

Non-neurological disease

Manifestations of cardiac, respiratory, endocrine or gastroin-testinal disease may be evident on general inspection. Do not overlook these as they may provide clues to the underlying aetiology of any neurological deficits.

Pronator drift

One arm will slowly pronate when the arms are in front and the eyes closed (**Figure 2.4**). This is a quite sensitive marker of an upper motor neuron lesion in the corticospinal tract.

Wasting and fasciculations

Wasting and fasciculations generally indicate lower motor neuron lesions:

- wasting: guttering of the interosseous muscles; flattening of the thenar or hypothenar eminences. This indicates a lower motor neuron lesion or chronic upper motor neuron lesion

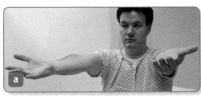

Figure 2.4 Testing for pronator drift. The patient holds their arms up, palms up and wide apart (a). On closing their eyes, a corticospinal tract lesion causes the arm to pronate and flex slightly at the elbow.

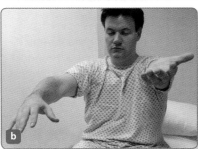

- fasciculations: spontaneous single muscle fibre contractions appearing as rippling of muscles. These indicate denervation and re-innervation of the neuromuscular junction, usually from lower motor neuron lesions

Abnormal posture

Abnormal postures may indicate distinct patterns of weakness:
- pyramidal distribution of weakness: there is greater weakness in the arm extensors than in the flexors, leading to a flexed elbow and wrist. This indicates an upper motor neuron lesion, e.g. cortical stroke
- dystonia: intermittent or constant contraction of agonist(s) and antagonist(s) muscles to produce an abnormally positioned body part

Dystonia

This is described by the body part affected:
- focal dystonia: only one body part is affected (e.g. torticollis from contraction of neck muscles)
- segmental: two or more adjacent parts affected.

It is classified by the underlying cause:
- primary: dystonia is the only clinical symptom
- heredodegenerative: e.g. Wilson's disease, Huntington's disease, neuroacanthocytosis
- secondary: hypoxic injury, stroke

Dystonia can occasionally cause rhythmic contractions, leading to a tremor resembling parkinsonism.

> ## Guiding principle
>
> 'Akinetic-rigid syndromes' is a term used to describe movement disorders characterised by reduced movement or increased rigidity. It largely refers to Parkinson's disease and Parkinson-plus disorders.

Abnormal movement

Movements may be reduced or excessive. Reduced movements include bradykinesia, which is a slowness or lack of movement. This is the hallmark of akinetic–rigid syndromes such as parkinsonism. Additional (excessive) movements include tremor, which is an involuntary rhythmic oscillation of a body part. It can be physiological or pathological, and is classified as a:
- resting tremor: present at rest, but may be exacerbated with distraction, e.g. Parkinson's disease
- action tremor
- psychogenic tremor: common. Usually it is variable, distractible, occurs inconsistently and may be entrainable (i.e. when the patient is asked to tap another limb at a different frequency from the tremor, the limb with the tremor then oscillates at the new frequency)

Action tremors

There are several different types of action tremor:
- postural: occurs when maintaining a posture, e.g. essential tremor, renal or liver disease
- kinetic: occurs during a voluntary movement
- intention: occurs at the end of target-directed movements, and is caused by cerebellar lesions
- task specific: occurs during specific tasks such as writing or playing a musical instrument

Tics

These are rapid and stereo-typed involuntary move-ments. They can be motor (e.g. eyelid movements or facial distortions) or vocal (e.g. coprolalia – expletives or socially inappropriate words) tics. Causes include Tourette's syndrome, neuroacanthocy-tosis and antipsychotics.

Chorea and athetosis

Chorea is involuntary, brief, jerky movements that flow continuously. Athetosis is slower involuntary movements that also flow. Distinguishing between them can be difficult and not usually clinically useful. Many patients have both: chore-athetoid movements.

> ### Clinical insight
>
> Rarer types of tremor include:
> - Holmes' tremor: this is an irregular, low-frequency tremor occurring at rest and with movement caused by lesions in the thalamus or midbrain
> - neuropathic tremor: this is usually from peripheral nerve demyelination
> - palatal tremor: seen in essential tremor (when it is associated with clicking in the ear from the eustachian tube), or in a lesion of Guillain–Mollaret's triangle (red nucleus–olives–dentate nucleus)

Myoclonus

This is involuntary and brief muscle twitching. It has confusingly disparate classifications according to the body part affected, clinical presentation or site of origin. More simply, it is described as positive or negative:
- positive myoclonus: sudden, brief, shock-like contraction of a muscle
- negative myoclonus: sudden, brief, shock-like loss of con-traction of a muscle (e.g. asterixis)

Gait

The gait can be largely symmetrical or asymmetrical, and gen-erally broad- or narrow-based. The patient may have difficulty initiating movements or turning.

Symmetrical abnormal gait

A symmetrical gait can be broad-based or narrow-based.

Broad-based

These include:

- cerebellar or vestibular lesions often cause an ataxia that produces a gait in which patients spread their legs widely, appear very unsteady and may seem reluctant to lift their feet at all. They will tend to veer towards the side of the lesion
- peripheral nerve sensory lesions cause a similar wide base, but patients may lift and slap both their feet more prominently

Narrow-based

These include:

- Parkinsonism usually presents with a slow shuffling gait. Patients are stooped forward and have a reduced arm swing. They struggle to initiate movements and take several steps to turn
- diffuse vascular disease may cause the marche à petits pas (march of a thousand steps, literally, 'walking with very small steps'), in which the narrow-based shuffling gait is accompanied by a more upright posture
- a myopathic gait appears waddling due to weakness in the proximal muscles

Asymmetrical gait

An asymmetrical gait can result from a wide range of problems:

- the hemiplegic gait is narrow based, although the affected leg will swing out to the side with a tilting movement of the hip during the movement
- foot drop: weakness of tibialis anterior from any cause will result in reduced ankle dorsiflexion and the characteristic floppy foot. Causes include L5 radiculopathy, common peroneal palsy and a cingulate gyrus lesion
- magnetic gait: this describes gait apraxia, in which the patient seems stuck to the floor. Causes include stroke and normal pressure hydrocephalus

The functional gait

This is inconsistent, variable and utilises inefficient movements (e.g. crouching movements).

2.3 General inspection

Objective

The objective of the general inspection is to identify any neurological syndromes or obvious weakness, deformity, abnormal posture or movement, wasting or fasciculations.

Approach

Patients strip to their undergarments, having been warned that they will be inspected closely.

Sequence

Use the following sequence:
1. ask the patient to undress, but to keep on their underwear
2. inspect the patient from front and from behind, noting the:
    - posture
    - skin colour, pigmentation, lesions, naevi
    - muscle bulk, wasting, fasciculations

Key differential diagnoses

There are innumerable syndromes with neurological manifestations, including:

- **Parkinson's disease:** patients have bradykinesia, hypomimic facies, tremor
- **Bell's palsy:** patients have lower facial nerve palsy and may be wearing an eye patch
- **acromegaly:** this is caused by a growth hormone-secreting pituitary tumour that results in excess growth of hands, feet and jaw; bitemporal hemianopia; and hypertension
- **myasthenia gravis:** antibodies directed against the neuromuscular junction cause muscle fatiguability; there is also bilateral ptosis and facial weakness, and obesity from steroid dependence
- **myotonic dystrophy type 1:** this is caused by a CTG trinucleotide expansion in the DMPK gene; patients have frontal balding, cataracts, muscle wasting, distal weakness, facial weakness and wasting, neck drop, cognitive impairment, cardiac conduction defects and cardiomyopathy, diabetes mellitus, dysphagia and chronic type 2 respiratory failure

- **Sturge–Weber syndrome:** this is caused by cerebral angioma, and patients have a port-wine stain over the distribution of V1
- **Charcot–Marie–Tooth diseases:** these are genetic syndromes causing peripheral nerve axonal or myelin disruption; a high-arched foot and claw toes
- **Huntington's disease:** patients display chorea–athetoid movements
- **dermatomyositis:** this is an inflammatory myopathy with characteristic skin changes: Gottron's sign, erythematous scaly lesions on the dorsum of the fingers; heliotrope rash, violaceous rash over the eyelids; shawl sign, a flat, erythematous rash over the chest in a V-shaped distribution
- **neurofibromatosis:** type 1 (von Recklinghausen's disease), there is an autosomal dominant mutation of the NF1 gene on chromosome 17q, and patients have neurofibromas, café-au-lait patches and phaeochromocytomas; type 2, there is an autosomal dominant mutation in the NF2 gene on chromosome 22, and patients have bilateral acoustic neuromas and meningiomas
- **tuberous sclerosis:** there is an autosomal dominant mutation of the tumour suppressor genes on chromosomes 9q or 16p, and patients have adenoma sebaceum (red papules on the face from angiofibromas), subungual fibromas, shagreen patches (elevated connective tissue naevi) and ashleaf patches (depigmented lesions best seen under a Wood's light)
- **Wilson's disease:** this is caused by an autosomal recessive mutation in the ATP7B gene encoding a copper-transporting protein, and patients have liver disease, movement disorder and Kayser–Fleischer rings (copper deposition in Descemet's membrane in the cornea)
- **ataxia telangiectasia:** this is the result of a mutation in the DNA repair gene ATM, and patients have ataxia and telangiectasias of the skin and eyes
- **spina bifida:** this is a range of developmental abnormalities of the neural tube resulting in abnormal spinal cord formation and hydrocephalus. There may be only subtle cutaneous signs over the sacral region such as a tuft of hair or dimple

What happens next?

After following the initial sequence described above, examine posture, movements and gait.

2.4 Abnormal posture and movements

Objective

The objective of the next stage is to identify any abnormal movements and to classify them.

Approach

Observe the gait without explicitly warning the patient as this can cause them to either involuntarily suppress abnormal movements or to manifest functional signs. Instead, during the history-taking part of the assessment, try to note any abnormal movements.

To further assess abnormal movements and to elicit latent signs, patients are usually asked to perform some specific tasks.

Equipment

For this part of the examination, pen and paper are required.

Sequence

The following sequence is used to assess abnormal movements and to elicit latent signs:

1. when taking the history, note whether there are any abnormal movements. Start at the patient's head and work down looking for a lack of movement or additional movements
2. note whether there is a general poverty of movement (i.e. reduced blink rate, hypomimia, slowed speech)
3. note:
- facial movements and head position
- arm positions and movements
- leg positions and movements
- any resting tremor
4. ask the patient to hold their hands out straight in front of them with their fingers spread out. Note any tremor
5. ask them to cock their wrists back and hold them there. Observe for asterixis

6. ask them to lift their arms out to the side and bring their fingertips together in front of their nose by bending their elbows and to hold that position (**Figure 2.5**). Note any dystonic posture or tremor

7. ask them to touch their forefinger to their thumb and to open and close that as fast and as fully as they can. Note any slowed speed or decreased amplitude

8. ask them to write a sentence and draw a spiral. Note any micrographia or oscillations that indicate a tremor

9. assess tone in their upper limbs (see Chapter 4), noting any cogwheeling or rigidity

Key differential diagnoses

Hypokinetic movement disorders

Patients in whom the main clinical findings are rigidity or reduced movement usually have one of the following disorders (listed with their key clinical features), with idiopathic Parkinson's disease being the most common.

Parkinson's disease

Parkinson's disease is idiopathic parkinsonism. Typically, there is unilateral onset and persistent asymmetry, rest tremor and slow progression of symptoms. The patient's initial response to L-dopa is good, but diminishes over time. Common symptoms include:

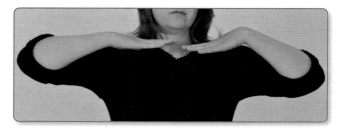

Figure 2.5 Testing for dystonic posture or tremor. The patient is asked to touch their fingers together in front of their chin. This can reveal dystonic posturing of the hand or arm, as seen here in the inability to fully straighten the left wrist.

- **bradykinesia:** reduced arm swing, slowed movements, reduced facial expression, slow to turn
- **resting tremor:** usually asymmetrical at onset in idiopathic Parkinson's disease
- **rigidity:** stiffness throughout range of movement of limbs, neck or trunk
- **anosmia:** this may have begun years previously
- **urinary symptoms:** if these are severe, this suggests multiple systems atrophy; the patient may have postural hypotension
- **restless legs syndrome:** again, it may pre-date the movement symptoms by decades
- **cognitive impairment:** if this is severe at the early stage, it may indicate dementia with Lewy bodies

Drug-induced parkinsonism

Often bilateral tremor. History of tremor-inducing medication.

Vascular parkinsonism

Often bilateral signs, lower limb predominant and a history of vascular risk factors.

> ## Clinical insight
>
> Dopa-responsive dystonia, or Segawa's disease, is a rare autosomal dominant inherited dystonia caused by mutation in the GTP cyclohydrolase 1 gene:
>
> - it usually presents in childhood or young adults
> - there may be mild parkinsonism; often, older patients are misdiagnosed with Parkinson's disease
> - L-dopa has a profound effect on the symptoms

Dementia with Lewy bodies

Dementia within 1 year of onset of parkinsonism, fluctuating cognition and hallucinations.

Multiple systems atrophy

Parkinsonism with cerebellar signs, orthostatic hypotension, urinary incontinence and preserved cognition.

Progressive supranuclear palsy

Rigidity of the trunk, early falls, dysarthria and cognitive decline.

Cortico-basal degeneration

Asymmetrical limb dyspraxia, rigidity and dystonia.

Clinical insight

Parkinsonism, slurred speech and either dystonia or tremor in a person under 40 years old should always make you think of Wilson's disease as the cause.

Wilson's disease is a disorder of excess copper storage in multiple organs, including the brain and is treated with copper chelation therapy.

Clinical insight

Drugs that commonly cause drug-induced tremor include:

- metaclopramide
- sodium valproate
- lithium
- tricyclic antidepressants
- beta-agnoists
- SSRIs
- diltiazem

Always review the medication history in patients with tremor.

Hyperkinetic movement disorders

Patients with abnormal, involuntary movements have their predominant movements defined as one of the following. Each is given with their most common differential diagnosis.

Tremor

Essential tremor, tremor of parkinsonism, dystonic tremor, cerebellar tremor (**Table 2.1**).

Dystonia

Primary dystonia, dopa-responsive dystonia, symptomatic dystonia (e.g. stroke, cerebral palsy), heredodegenerative dystonia (e.g. Wilson's disease, Huntington's disease).

Myoclonus

Epileptic myoclonus (occuring as part of an epileptic

Feature	Parkinson's disease	Essential tremor
Prevalence	Less common	Very common
At rest	Worst	Less severe
On action	Suppressed	Severe
Family history	Rare	Very common
Effect of alcohol	None	Alleviates
Head tremor	Almost never	Common

Table 2.1 Comparison of the tremor of Parkinson's disease and essential tremor

syndrome), secondary myoclonus (trauma, hypoxia), symptomatic myoclonus [e.g. Friedreich's ataxia, Wilson's disease, Huntington's disease, Creutzfeldt–Jakob disease (CJD), dementia] metabolic or toxic causes (e.g. renal failure, liver failure, tricyclic antidepressants, morphine, SSRIs, antipyschotics).

Chorea

Inherited (e.g. Huntington's disease, Wilson's disease, Friedreich's ataxia, tuberous sclerosis), acquired (e.g. stroke, drugs, thyrotoxicosis, CJD, post-streptococcal).

Tics

Gilles de la Tourette's syndrome, Wilson's disease, autism, antipsychotics.

What happens next?

The next stage is to examine the patient's gait.

2.5 Assessing gait

Objective

The objective of this stage is to assess the co-ordinated sensory, planning and motor skills involved in walking.

Approach

Observe the patient walking and performing a few movements.

Equipment

No equipment is required for this part of the examination.

Sequence

The following sequence is used:

1. ask the patient to stand as able

Clinical insight

Examining shoes in patients with abnormal gait can be informative:

- worn-in shoes are good indicators of the usual gait pattern and may confirm that the observed abnormal gait has been consistently present for some time

- shoes with a normal pattern of wear may suggest the gait dysfunction is intermittent. This does not exclude organic pathology but could suggest a functional disorder or deliberate malingering

2. ask them to put their feet together and close their eyes. Ensure they do not fall. This is Romberg's test. If the patient sways markedly and loses their balance, the test is positive and indicates loss of proprioception

3. ask the patient to walk to the other end of the room. Observe the stride length, pattern, width of base, dorsiflexion of the ankle, speed, turning and arm swing

4. ask them to turn and come back

5. ask the patient to walk away again, heel to toe; if they manage this, have them walk heel to toe backwards

6. ask the patient to walk on their toes, then their heels

7. ask them to squat down and stand up without touching the floor

8. test for retropulsion by standing behind them and pulling their shoulders towards you. See how many steps they take to steady themselves, but do not let them fall

Key differential diagnoses

These include the following:

Parkinsonism

Patients have a slow, shuffling gait, reduced arm swing and take many steps to turn; they may take several steps to avoid falling on retropulsion. This results from basal ganglia dysfunction.

Hemiplegic gait

Patients walk with an extended hip and ankle that swings out to the side. It is commonly caused by hemispheric stroke.

Scissoring

There is bilateral extended hips and ankles from a spastic paraparesis. Causes include multiple sclerosis and anoxic brain injury.

Ataxia

This is covered in more detail in Chapter 6; it appears as a broad-based unsteady gait. Broad categories of cause include:

- sensory: from loss of proprioceptive input – Romberg's positive; causes include numerous peripheral neuropathies or posterior column lesions (e.g. alcohol, cord compression, vitamin B_{12} deficiency)
- cerebellar: from a lesion there – Romberg's negative; patients fall to the side of the lesion and have poor heel-to-toe walking; causes include alcohol, stroke, cerebellar degeneration, posterior fossa tumour
- midline or vermal cerebellar lesions: often cause an unsteadiness of the head, neck and trunk even while sitting or standing with the eyes open. Patients will struggle to stand with their feet together even with their eyes open

Antalgic gait

Patients struggle to bear weight on the affected leg and shuffle along. There is a wide range of causes from orthopaedic to rheumatological. Nerve root lesions are typically very painful and may restrict movement.

Myopathy

Proximal myopathy may cause a waddling appearance and patients will struggle to squat and rise.

Weak toe walking

This is caused by a weak gastrocnemius.

Poor heel walking

This is caused by a weak tibialis anterior.

What happens next?

Referral to a neurologist with a specialist interest in movement disorders is recommended for all patients with parkinsonism, dystonia, unexplained myoclonus or athetosis or chorea. MRI is indicated to investigate cerebellar lesions or suspected spinal cord pathology.

2.6 System summary

The examination of gait and general inspection is summarised in **Table 2.2**.

Inspection	Observe during history
	Expose and inspect
Abnormal posture and movements	Note position of: head, neck, trunk, limbs
	Observe for: poverty of movement; tremor, tics, chorea, athetosis, myoclonus
	Observe: outstretched arms; cocked wrists; fingers touching under nose; open and closing finger movements; writing; spiral drawing
	Check tone in arms
Gait	Stand patient up
	Romberg's test
	Walk to end of room and back
	Heel to toe
	Walk on toes
	Walk on heels
	Squat
	Retropulsion

Table 2.2 The key aspects of general inspection and examining the gait

Head and neck (cranial nerves)

3.1 Objectives

Examination of the cranial nerves is a vital skill for students and junior doctors. The principles are identical to any other portion of the neurological examination but many students and physicians find this part daunting. It need not be so.

This chapter is on the 'head and neck' rather than on 'cranial nerves' to remind the clinician that the neurological assessment includes not only the nerves themselves but also the whole neuroaxis from the muscle or sensory endings, neuromuscular junction, peripheral cranial nerve fibres and brainstem nuclei to the higher centres.

As with other parts of the examination, the key principles are to:
- detect abnormal signs
- localise any lesions
- identify potential pathogenic processes

3.2 Anatomy and physiology review

Relevant anatomy, physiology, connections, functions and arterial supply of the 12 cranial nerves are summarised in **Tables 3.1–3.3**. The nerves exit the skull through the exit formina (**Figure 3.1**); the location of their nuclei in the brainstem are shown in **Figure 3.2**.

CN I: the olfactory nerve

The olfactory nerve:
- is a purely sensory nerve
- runs in the olfactory groove
- is prone to damage from head injury

CN II: the optic nerve

Testing the visual field produces characteristic abnormal findings depending on the location of the lesion (**Figure 3.3**).

Cranial nerve	Motor innervation	Sensory input	Autonomic component	Brainstem nuclei
I Olfactory	–	Bipolar sensory cells of olfactory epithelium	–	–
II Optic	–	Axons from retinal ganglion cells	–	Thalamus Midbrain
III Oculomotor	Levator palpabrae superioris Superior rectus Medial rectus Inferior rectus Inferior oblique	–	Preganglionic para-sympathetic fibres to sphincter of iris (constriction and acco-mmodation)	Parasym-pathetic Edinger–Westphal nucleus Motor Oculomotor nucleus
IV Trochlear	Superior oblique	–	–	Pons
VI Abducens	Lateral rectus	–	–	Junction of pons and medulla

Table 3.1 Cranial nerve supply to the nose and eyes

The optic nerve:
- is a purely sensory nerve originating as retinal ganglion cells
- passes through the optic canal (**Figure 3.1**)
- contributes the afferent limb of the pupillary reflex (**Figure 3.4**)

CN III, IV and VI: the eye muscle nerves
CN III, IV and VI:
- control eye movements (**Figure 3.5**)
- IV and VI are purely motor

Cranial nerve	Motor innervation	Sensory input	Autonomic component	Brainstem nuclei
V Trigeminal	Muscles of mastication; tensor tympani	Mucous membranes of mouth, nose and paranasal air sinuses and skin of head and face	Ciliary, pterygopalatine, otic and submandibular ganglia	Motor nuclei in pons Sensory in pons, brainstem and spinal cord dorsal horn nuclei
VII Facial	Muscles of facial expression Stapedius muscle of middle ear	Taste fibres from anterior 2/3 of the tongue Sensory fibres from external ear	Parasympathetic secretomotor fibres to sublingual and submandibular salivary glands, lacrimal gland and nasal mucosa	Motor in pons Sensory in medulla
VIII Vestibulo-cochlear	–	Bipolar spiral ganglion cells Vestibular fibres	–	Cochlear nuclei in medulla Vestibular nuclei in medulla and pons

Table 3.2 Cranial nerve supply to the face and ears

- III is motor with a parasympathetic component of CN III mediating the efferent limb of the pupillary reflex via the ciliary ganglion (**Figure 3.4**)
- III innervates all eye muscles (inferior oblique, inferior rectus, superior rectus, medial rectus and levator palpabrae superioris) except superior oblique (IV) and lateral rectus (VI)
- pass through the cavernous sinus and the superior orbital fissure and can be involved in a lesion in either (**Figure 3.1**)

Cranial nerve	Motor innervation	Sensory input	Autonomic component	Brainstem nuclei
IX Glosso-pharyngeal	Stylo-pharyngeus muscle	Pharynx and posterior 1/3 of the tongue	Para-sympathetic secretomotor fibres to the parotid gland	Motor in medulla Para-sympathetic in pons
X Vagus	Muscles of larynx, pharynx and palate involved in speech	Larynx Portion of external auditory meatus Viscerosensory from gastrointestinal tract, lungs, heart and aortic arch	Para-sympathetic innervation of bronchi, bronchioles, atria of heart, liver, gallbladder, pancreas, oesophagus, stomach, gut (to colonic flexure) and kidneys	Motor, sensory and para-sympathetic in medulla
XI Accessory	Cranial roots: muscles of palate, larynx and pharynx Spinal roots: trapezius and sternocleido-mastoid muscles	–	–	Cranial root in medulla Spinal root in spinal cord
XII Hypoglossal	Muscles of the tongue	–	–	Medulla

Table 3.3 The lower cranial nerves

CN V: the trigeminal nerve
The trigeminal nerve is:
- a large nerve with ophthalmic (V_1), maxillary (V_2) and man-dibular divisions (V_3)

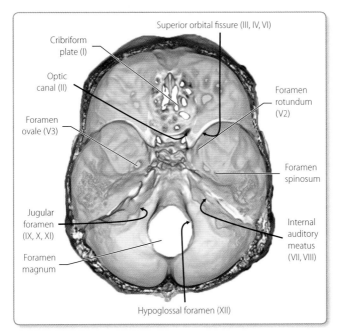

Figure 3.1 The skull foramina.

- mixed motor, sensory and autonomic (**Figure 3.6**)
- Each division courses to a different area of the head and face (**Figure 3.6**):
- V_1 passes through the cavernous sinus and carries sensation from the forehead and upper eyelid and nose
- V_2 passes through the foramen rotundum and carries sensation from around the cheekbones and from the sinus and nose
- V_3 passes through the infratemporal fossa and carries sensation from the lower jaw and innervates the muscles of mastication

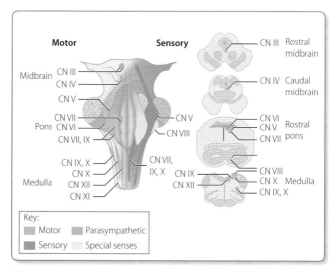

Figure 3.2 Brainstem localisation of cranial nerve nuclei.

CN VII: the facial nerve

The facial nerve:
- is a mixed motor, sensory and autonomic nerve
- controls the muscles of facial expression, stapedius muscle of the inner ear (problems with which lead to hyperacusis), taste from the anterior two-thirds of the tongue and innervation of the lacrimal gland
- passes through the internal auditory meatus/cerebellopontine angle (**Figure 3.1**) and the parotid gland (**Figure 3.7**)

Clinical insight

Think 'face, ear, taste, tear' to remember the basic functions of CN VII.

CN VIII: the vestibulocochlear nerve

The vestibulocochlear nerve:
- is purely sensory
- mediates hearing and vestibular balance

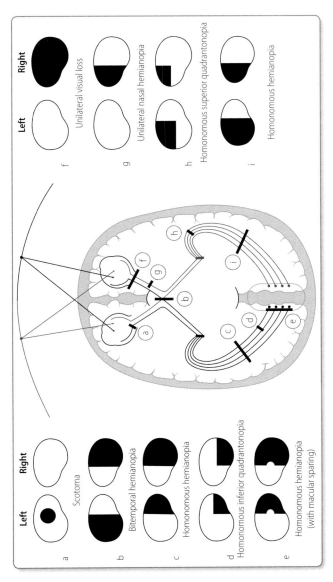

Figure 3.3 Localising visual field defects.

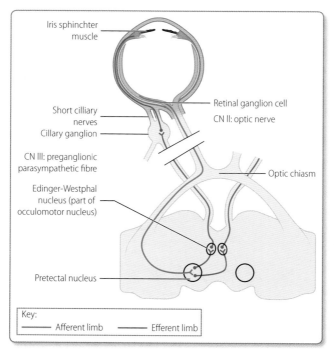

Figure 3.4 The pupillary reflex arc involves CN II (afferent limb) and CN III (efferent limb) at the level of the midbrain.

- passes through the cerebellopontine angle with the facial nerve

CN IX: the glossopharyngeal nerve

The glossopharyngeal nerve:
- is mixed motor, sensory and autonomic
- passes through the jugular foramen (**Figures 3.1** and **3.8**)
- elevates the pharynx and larynx
- carries sensation from the pharynx and posterior one-third of the tongue

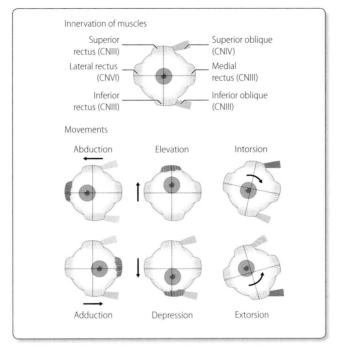

Figure 3.5 Cranial innervation of eye muscles and eye movements. The tendon of the superior oblique muscle loops through the trochlear nerve, changing the direction of muscle movement. As a result, activation of the superior oblique rotates the pupil inward toward the nose and downward (intorsion). The inferior oblique rotates the pupil outward and upward (extorsion).

- carries parasympathetic fibres to the parotid
- carries sensory information from the carotid sinus and carotid bodies

CN X: the vagus nerve
The vagus nerve:
- innervates some of the muscles of speech

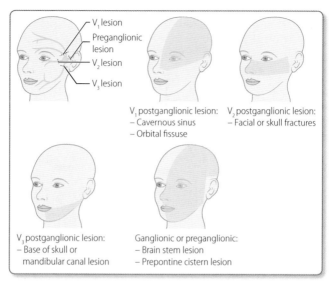

Figure 3.6 The trigeminal nerve. The pattern of sensory changes points towards which part of the nerve is damaged.

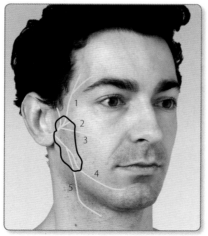

Figure 3.7 The facial nerve passes through the parotid gland. Tumours here can cause lower motor neuron facial nerve lesions. 1, Temporal branch; 2, zygomatic branch; 3, buccal branches; 4, marginal mandibular branch; 5, cervical branch.

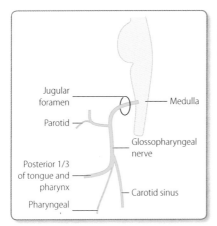

Figure 3.8 The glossopharyngeal nerve mediates the afferent limb of the gag reflex.

- carries much of the parasympathetic innervation of the chest and abdominal cavity
- passes through the jugular foramen (**Figure 3.1**) and over the hilum of the lung

CN XI: the accessory nerve

The accessory nerve:
- is purely motor
- has cranial and spinal roots
- passes through the foramen magnum and jugular foramen (**Figures 3.1** and **3.9**)
- cranial roots are essentially a caudal portion of the vagus
- spinal roots innervate trapezius and sternocleidomastoid

> ### Clinical insight
>
> Any lesion in the hilum can cause a phrenic nerve (a branch of the vagus) palsy.

CN XII: the hypoglossal nerve

The hypoglossal nerve:
- is purely motor
- passes through the hypoglossal foramen (**Figure 3.1**)
- innervates the muscles of the tongue

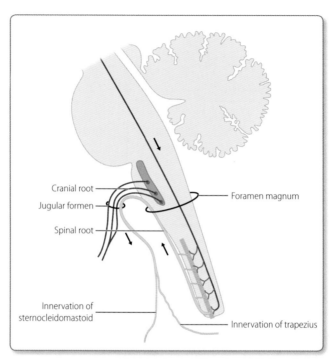

Figure 3.9 Accessory nerve. The spinal roots pass up through the foramen magnum and join the cranial root, which then branches off to run with the vagus nerve. The remainder forms the main body of the accessory nerve and innervates the trapezius and sternocleidomastoid muscles.

The pupillary reflexes

The pupillary reflexes include:
- the light reflex to adjust retinal exposure
- the accommodation reflex to adjust focus
- vergence to co-ordinate binocular focus

Direct reflex

The afferent limb of the light reflex consists of the retina, optic nerve, optic chiasm, optic tract, superior colliculus and

Edinger–Westphal nuclei in the midbrain (**Figure 3.4**). The efferent limb consists of the Edinger–Westphal nucleus, preganglionic parasympathetic fibres in the superficial oculomotor nerve, the ciliary ganglion and the sphincter muscles of the iris and ciliary body. The neurons in the Edinger–Westphal nucleus send the efferent signal to both oculomotor nerves, meaning that shining a light into one eye will constrict the pupils of both (the consensual reflex).

Accommodation reflex

A normal accommodation reflex is for the pupils to constrict as the patient focuses on near vision. The afferent limb of this reflex begins with the frontal eye fields in the frontal lobes, rather than the optic nerve. The efferent path is the same as the direct light reflex.

> ### Clinical insight
>
> Afferent refers to the sensory or input portion of a reflex. Efferent refers to the output or effector portion of the reflex. Remember that A comes before E and, in a reflex, the Afferent limb comes before the Efferent limb.

3.3 Clinical features and pathophysiology

Relevant abnormal findings, corresponding location of lesions and common cranial nerve and brainstem syndromes are summarised in **Tables 3.4** and **3.5**. The key pathological findings are as follows.

CN II
Swollen optic disc
This is an elevated disc with blurred margins, venous engorgement and loss of venous pulsation.

Pathophysiology
This results from either papilloedema or papillitis:
- papilloedema: swollen disc caused by raised intracranial pressure; pressure on the retinal vessels and nerves can cause irreversible loss of vision (late)
- papillitis: swollen disc caused by inflammation; retinal or optic nerve inflammation causes acute visual loss (early) and pain on moving the eyes

Syndrome	Cranial nerves involved	Location of lesion	Typical causes	Clinical features
Bell's palsy	VII	VII nerve	Idiopathic	Unilateral lower motor neuron facial nerve weakness, hyperacusis, loss of taste, dry eyes
Tolosa–Hunt syndrome	III, IV, VI (V1)	Polyneuropathy	Idiopathic inflammation	Unilateral orbital pain over weeks
Cavernous sinus syndrome	III, IV, VI (V1)	Cavernous sinus	Carotid dissection, carotid aneurysm, thrombophlebitis of sinus, infection of sinus	Progressive ophthalmoplegia, painful diplopia, exophthalmos
Ramsay–Hunt syndrome	VII (V)	VII nerve	Herpes zoster	Acute unilateral facial palsy following ear pain with vesicles in auditory meatus
Jugular foramen syndrome	IX, X, XI	Jugular foramen	Glomus tumour, meningioma, acoustic neuroma, metastases, trauma	Unilateral hoarseness, loss of gag reflex, uvula deviates, dysphagia, sternocleidomastoid and trapezius weakness
Cerebellopontine angle	V, VII, VIII	Cerebellopontine angle	Acoustic neuroma, lipoma, vascular malformation, metastases	Hearing loss, tinnitus, vertigo, facial numbness
Bulbar palsy	Bilateral lower motor neuron X, XI, XII	Nuclei of affected nerves or peripheral nerves	Guillain–Barré syndrome, motor neuron disease, sarcoidosis	Dysphagia, dysarthria, loss of gag reflex, tongue fasciculations
Pseudobulbar palsy	Bilateral upper motor neuron X, XI, XII	Corticobulbar tracts, supranuclear lesions	Motor neuron disease	Dysphagia, dysarthria, exaggerated gag and jaw reflex, pseudobulbar affect, slow spastic tongue

Table 3.4 Cranial nerve syndromes

Brainstem syndrome	Cranial nerves nuclei involved	Location of lesion	Artery affected	Clinical features
Medial medulla syndrome	XI	Medial medulla	Distal vertebral artery	CL: arm and leg weakness, loss of PP and Vib IL: tongue weakness
Wallenberg syndrome (lateral medulla syndrome)	VIII, IX, X	Lateral medulla	Distal vertebral ± PICA	CL: loss of PP, Temp IL: limb ataxia, loss of PP, Temp, Horner syndrome Vertigo, nystagmus, nausea, vomiting, hoarseness, dysphagia
Medial pons	VI, VII	Medial pons	Basilar perforators	CL: arm, leg and facial weakness, ataxia IL: abducens weakness INO Paralysis of conjugate gaze to side of infarction
Lateral pons	V, VII, VIII	Lateral pons	AICA	CL: loss of sensation on body IL: limb ataxia, facial weakness, Horner syndrome, deafness, tinnitus Vertigo, nystagmus
Weber syndrome	III, VII	Midbrain peduncle	PCA	CL: face, arm and leg weakness IL: medial rectus weakness, mydriasis Impaired vertical gaze
Midbrain tegmentum	III	Midbrain tegmentum	PCA	CL: limb ataxia, choreoathetosis, hemiballism IL: medial rectus weakness, mydriasis Impaired vertical gaze

Table 3.5 Brainstem syndromes. AICA, anterior inferiorcerebellar artery. CL, contralateral. IL, ipsilateral. INO, internuclear ophthalmoplegia. PCA, posterior communicating artery. PICA, posterior inferior cerebellar artery. PP, pin prick sensation. Temp, temperature sensation. Vib, vibration sense

Pale disc

A pale white colour suggests optic atrophy from any cause.

Pathophysiology

The causes of a pale disc include retinal or nerve head ischaemia or a chronic phase of optic neuritis leading to degeneration of the retinal ganglion cells.

Diabetic retinopathy

There is rubeosis (blood vessel formation over the iris), cataracts and other key features:
- proliferative changes: new blood vessel formation, haemorrhages, scars, retinal detachment
- non-proliferative changes: microaneurysms, dot and blot haemorrhages, hard (lipid) and soft (ischaemia) exudates

Staging of diabetic retinopathy is shown in **Table 3.6**.

Pathophysiology

This is multifactorial. Chronic hyperglycaemia leads to new vessel formation; these vessels are fragile and prone to bleeding.

Hypertensive retinopathy

This is graded as shown in **Table 3.7**.

Pathophysiology

This results from systemic hypertension, which causes accelerated arterial sclerosis and the above changes. Changes can occur slowly over years with chronic hypertension or acutely over days with malignant hypertension.

Central retinal artery occlusion

This is a rapid, painless, loss of vision with a milky-white fundus and thin arteries.

Pathophysiology

Occlusion or inflammation of the central retinal artery, causes nerve fibre ischaemia. Commonly, this arises from carotid artery stenosis (i.e. amaurosis fugax).

Stage	Features
1	Non-proliferative/background retinopathy: microaneurysms, hard exudates, dot–blot haemorrhages
2	Maculopathy: changes occur in the macula
3	Proliferative retinopathy: neovascularisation, vitreous haemorrhages, retinal detachment

Table 3.6 Staging diabetic retinopathy

Grade	Features
1	Silver wiring (sclerotic vessels appear silvery)
2	Grade 1 plus marked deflection of veins as they cross arteries (arteriovenous nipping)
3	Grade 2 plus flame haemorrhages and soft and hard exudates
4	Grade 3 plus papilloedema

Table 3.7 Grading of hypertensive retinopathy

Central retinal vein thrombosis

There are twisted retinal veins with widespread haemorrhages and an 'apocalyptic blood and thunder' appearance.

Pathophysiology

Thrombosis from any cause in the major draining vein from the retina cause engorged veins, oedema, haemorrhages and variable visual loss. A narrow exit of the vein through the lamina cribrosa predisposes to venous stasis and thrombosis.

Hemianopia

This is a loss of a portion of the visual field. It differs from retinal scotomas in that the defect persists when either eye is closed in turn.

Pathophysiology

Figure 3.3 elaborates on localising visual field defects. In general, a homonymous hemianopia indicates a retrochiasmal lesion.

Pupils

Dilated pupil

This results from a failure to constrict to light. The following can be distinguished:

- normal accommodation: relative afferent papillary defect (RAPD) (i.e. retinal or optic nerve disease; **Figure 3.10**)
- slow accommodation: Holmes–Adie pupil
- failure of accommodation: IIIrd nerve palsy or drug effect.

Pathophysiology

RAPD results from a failure to stimulate the light reflex on the affected side owing to retinal or optic nerve pathology, such as optic neuritis in multiple sclerosis. The affected pupil will constrict via the consensual reflex when light is shone in other eye. A Holmes–Adie pupil is tonically dilated from degeneration of the ciliary ganglion. It will accommodate slowly. A IIIrd nerve palsy will cause ptosis and the eye will be depressed and abducted ('down and out'). If there is a 'surgical cause' (i.e. posterior communicating artery aneurysm), there will be pupillary involvement: a large unreactive pupil (**Figures 3.11** and **3.13a**).

Constricted pupil

This results from a failure to dilate in low light. The following can be distinguished:

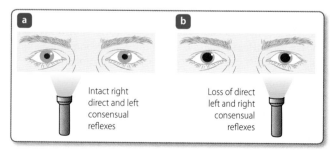

a   Intact right direct and left consensual reflexes

b   Loss of direct left and right consensual reflexes

Figure 3.10 A left relative afferent papillary defect. (a) The left pupil constricts on shining a torch in the right eye, indicating an intact afferent and efferent limb. (b) The left pupil is larger when the torch is directly shone on it, indicating a lesion in the afferent limb.

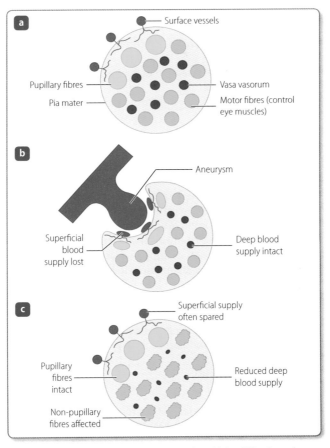

Figure 3.11 Medical and surgical IIIrd nerve palsies. (a) Small blood vessels on the surface of the pia mater supply the pupillar fibres of CN III, which lie superficial to the motor fibres. The vasa vasorum supplies blood to the motor nerve fibres in the deeper region of CN III. (b) External compression of the nerve from a mass lesion involves the superficial blood supply early in the course of the disease, so the pupillary fibres are affected and there is a dilated pupil: a 'surgical' third nerve palsy. (c) Injury to the deep blood supply from toxic or metabolic disorders, such as diabetes or hypertension, affects the motor fibres but often spares the superficial blood supply to the pupillary fibres: a 'medical' third nerve palsy.

- unreactive to light with normal accommodation: Argyll Robertson pupil
- unreactive to light with no accommodation: likely drug effect
- small with a sluggish reaction to light is common in elderly (senile meiosis)
- small, sluggish, ptosis, anhidrosis: Horner's syndrome (**Figure 3.12**)

Pathophysiology

Senile meiosis is a common cause. Argyll Robertson pupils are rare but indicate a midbrain lesion; causes include diabetes and syphilis. Horner's syndrome is caused by a lesion in the sympathetic supply to the eye, causing tonic constriction. Lesions can be in the hypothalamus, medulla, cervical cord, superior cervical ganglion or carotid artery. Stroke is a common cause in the central nervous system; a Pancoast tumour in the apex of the lung is an important peripheral cause. In young people, it suggests carotid artery dissection (**Figure 3.12**).

CN III, IV, VI
Ptosis

Ptosis is weakness of the levator palpebrae superioris (eyelid muscle), resulting in drooping of the eyelid. It can be partial, full, unilateral or bilateral.

Pathophysiology

This can be:

- bilateral, in which there is likely to be primary muscle or neuromuscular junction disease (e.g. myopathy, myasthenia gravis)
- unilateral, owing to a lesion of the IIIrd nerve or nuclei. If painful, the eye is 'down and out' and the ptosis is accompanied by a large unreactive pupil, assume that there is an expanding aneurysm until proven otherwise. Diabetic infarction of the IIIrd nerve may spare the pupil (**Figure 3.11**)

Down and out

In primary gaze, the eye appears to be depressed and abducted.

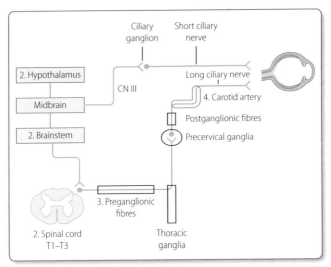

Figure 3.12 Localisation of Horner's syndrome. Horner's syndrome (ptosis, miosis and anhydrosis) can be caused by a lesion at various points between the hypothalamus and the carotid artery. 1, A lesion in CN III causes pupillary dilation rather than a Horner's syndrome. 2, Lesions from the hypothalamus to the spinal cord can cause a Horner's syndrome, as can lesions in the apex of the lung (3) or carotid artery (4).

Pathophysiology
This indicates IIIrd nerve palsy. Unopposed action from the lateral rectus muscle (CN VI) and superior oblique (CN IV) cause the eye to be depressed and abducted (**Figure 3.13**).

Tilted head
The patient holds their head at an angle to avoid diplopia. This may be subtle and the patient may not be aware of it.

Pathophysiology
The patient's posture can be indicative as the head tilts away from the side of the affected IVth nerve. This compensates for the failure of the superior oblique to intort the eye.

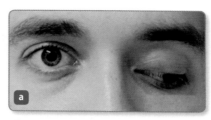

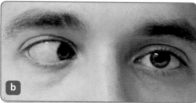

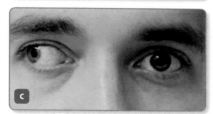

Figure 3.13 (a) Left IIIrd nerve palsy. (b) Left VIth nerve palsy. (c) Internuclear ophthalmoplegia on attempted right lateral gaze. Left eye fails to adduct owing to a lesion in the left medial longitudinal fasciculus. The left eye will adduct on accommodation.

Lateral rectus palsy

In lateral rectus palsy, the affected eye appears slightly adducted. There is horizontal diplopia, and weakness in eye abduction.

Pathophysiology

This results from failure of the lateral rectus because of VIth nerve palsy, which leaves the eye partially adducted owing to unopposed action of CN III and IV. This is a false localising sign as the VIth nerve can be affected from any cause of raised intracranial pressure since the nerve passes over the clivus (depression in the base of the skull), where it is vulnerable to compression (**Figure 3.13**).

CN V
Absent corneal reflex
This is a failure of the blink reflex on stimulation of the cornea. Stimulation on one side should normally provoke blink on both sides.

Pathophysiology
This is due to a lesion in CN V, which will cause loss of the afferent limb of the reflex arc with the loss of blink on the affected side and on the contralateral side. The efferent limb of the arc is mediated by the VIIth nerve. A lesion in the VIIth nerve results in the loss of blink on the affected side but preserved blink on the contralateral side.

Trigeminal neuralgia
This is a brief stabbing, shooting, electric shock-like pain in the distribution of the trigeminal nerve. It is provoked by touching the face, chewing or drinking.

Pathophysiology
The neuralgia is caused by a lesion in the trigeminal nerve or nuclei. It can be idiopathic or it can be secondary to an ectatic superior cerebellar artery irritating the trigeminal nerve root.

Brisk jaw jerk
Jaw jerk is usually mild or absent. A brisk jaw jerk suggests an upper motor neuron (UMN) lesion affecting the trigeminal nerve nuclei.

Pathophysiology
There is disinhibition of the local reflex circuitry in the brainstem because of degeneration of UMNs. This is caused by any UMN lesion, e.g. stroke, but is often seen in the context of motor neuron disease.

CN VII
Facial asymmetry
In facial asymmetry, there is a flattened nasolabial fold, down-turned mouth and there may be weakness of the eyelid and a loss of forehead wrinkles.

Pathophysiology

This is caused by unilateral cortical lesions (e.g. stroke), which spare the forehead and eyelid as the brainstem nuclei to these receive bilateral cortical innervation. Unilateral brainstem or lower motor neuron (LMN) lesions involve the forehead and eyelid. Bell's palsy (idiopathic inflammation of the facial nerve) is usually dramatic in the apparent weakness.

> ### Clinical insight
>
> Patients with Bell's palsy frequently perceive themselves as having the abnormality on the opposite side of the face to the one actually affected. An examining doctor may be led astray by listening to the patient telling them which side is affected. Patients also often report a subjective change in facial sensation, despite the Vth nerve not being involved and a normal Vth nerve examination. This may be due to a change in muscle tone with the facial nerve palsy.
>
> Always record what you see as well as what the patient says – even when they do not agree.

CN VIII
Conductive deafness

There is a subjective loss of hearing on the affected side. No vibration is heard in the affected ear when a tuning fork is moved in front of the ear in Rinne's test (Rinne negative). Vibration is heard louder in the affected ear in Weber's test.

Pathophysiology

In the presence of middle or external ear pathology (e.g. wax), this results from air conduction in front of the ear in Rinne's test not being transmitted to the cochlear nerve, but conduction through the skull is better so is heard better in the affected ear.

Sensorineural deafness

There is subjective hearing loss on the affected side, vibration is heard in the affected ear when the tuning fork is moved in front of the ear in Rinne's test (Rinne positive) and vibration is heard louder in the unaffected ear in Weber's test.

Pathophysiology

This is caused by a lesion in the central components of hearing (e.g. acoustic neuroma), which results in failure of both air- and bone-conducted sound equally in Rinne's test and preservation of hearing in the normal ear in Weber's test.

CN IX, X
Displaced uvula
The uvula deviates towards the normal side on saying 'Ah' in unilateral Xth nerve palsy.

Pathophysiology

This results from a lesion in the vagus nerve causing weakness of the muscles elevating the soft palate. An intact contralateral vagus pulls the soft palate towards the normal side. In bilateral lesions, the uvula will not elevate at all.

Abnormal gag reflex
A lesion in the afferent limb (glossopharyngeal) or efferent limb (vagus) results in loss of the gag reflex. An exaggerated gag reflex, in which minimal stimulation causes violent gag, occurs in UMN lesions affecting the IXth or Xth nuclei (e.g. motor neuron disease).

Pathophysiology

A unilateral lesion in the glossopharyngeal nerve causes loss of sensation and loss of the motor component of the reflex on both sides. A unilateral lesion in the vagus nerve causes intact sensation of the reflex, an absent motor component of the reflex on the affected side and a present motor component of the reflex on the unaffected side.

Laryngeal nerve palsy
There is hoarseness in unilateral laryngeal nerve palsy. With bilateral lesions, there is aphonia or respiratory distress.

Pathophysiology

The laryngeal nerves are branches of the vagus nerves. They course down into the thorax, through the mediastinum and back up into the neck. The right laryngeal nerve is vulnerable to trauma from thyroid surgery. The left laryngeal is prone to compression from mediastinal tumours.

CN XI
Weakness of trapezius or sternocleidomastoid
Patients present with weakness of shoulder elevation (trapezius) or head rotation (sternocleidomastoid muscle turns the head away).

Pathophysiology
Unilateral weakness indicates neck trauma or a mass in the jugular foramen. Bilateral weakness indicates generalised peripheral neuropathy, muscle disease or motor neuron disease.

CN XII
Slow and spastic tongue
Patients have a small, immobile tongue; this may be associated with dysarthria or dysphagia.

Pathophysiology
There is an UMN lesion affecting the XIIth nerve nuclei, which results in increased tone and weakness of the tongue. It eventually wastes. Common causes include motor neuron disease and stroke.

Wasted tongue
Unilateral LMN lesions of the XIIth nerve cause the tongue to deviate towards the weaker side on protrusion. Wasting and fasciculations occur secondary to denervation.

Pathophysiology
Bilateral lesions can occur from motor neuron disease or Guillain–Barré syndrome. Unilateral lesions result from motor neuron disease, tumours in the cervical region or lymphadenopathy.

3.4 General observations

Objective
The objective is to identify any gross abnormality of the head or neck from the bedside. Specifically think of:
- syndromes (e.g. neurofibromatosis, dermatomyositis, shingles, myotonic dystrophy, parkinsonism, Wilson's disease, Sturge–Weber syndrome)

- signs of non-neurological disease
- signs of generalised neurological disease
- head posture
- facial muscle tone, symmetry and ptosis
- nystagmus
- photo- or phonophobia

Approach
The patient removes their outer garments.

Equipment
You will need an ophthalmoscope, Snellen chart, otoscope, pen torch, Neurotips, tuning fork, tongue depressor, orange stick/throat swab, tendon hammer and cotton wool swab for the remainder of the examination.

Sequence
Use the following as a guide:
1. inspect the patient from the front and behind
2. look specifically for the features above and for any other signs expected from the history
3. look for any scars, evidence of head injury or surgery to the head or neck
4. test for neck stiffness

> **Clinical insight**
>
> Patients often struggle to understand every instruction of this examination, so make sure your instructions are unambiguous and precise. Mirroring the required movements or positions yourself is often useful.

Key differential diagnoses
See **Table 3.8** for key findings on general inspection.

What happens next?
The remainder of the neurological examination follows. The cranial nerves can be conveniently assessed in groups based on the part of the head being examined; think 'nose, eyes, face, ears, mouth and neck'.

Carry out a general physical examination.

3.5 The nose (CN I)

Objective
The objective is to identify and document any change or loss in the patient's sense of smell.

Approach
Formal testing is rarely performed or informative. However, particularly after head injury, the loss of sense of smell can have a significant impact on some patients and it is not infrequently a source of compensation claims.

Equipment
No equipment is required for informal or screening assessment. Three or four non-noxious smells should be presented to the patient if formally testing smell, e.g. orange peel, coffee beans, perfume and tobacco.

Finding	Key differential
Meningism (neck stiffness, photophobia, phonophobia)	Meningitis, encephalitis, subarachnoid haemorrhage, migraine
Head drop	Myopathy or myotonic dystrophy
Head rotated	Torticollis
Head tilted	VIth nerve palsy, skew deviation
Hemiplegia	Cortical or brainstem stroke
Generalised wasting	Myopathy, motor neuron disease, myelopathy
Ptosis	Congenital, myasthenia gravis, Miller Fisher syndrome, IIIrd nerve palsy
Facial asymmetry	Stroke, Bell's palsy, multiple sclerosis, migraine

Table 3.8 Key findings on general inspection

Sequence

Use the following sequence:
1. ask: 'Any change in your sense of smell or taste?'
5. for more formal assessment, present three or four easily recognisable scents to the patient (see above). Occlude each nostril in turn and ask the patient if they (1) smell anything and (2) recognise the smell

Key differential diagnoses

Acquired anosmia is common and generally benign. Common causes include upper respiratory tract infection and age-related loss; rare causes are parkinsonism and frontal lobe mass (unilateral).

What happens next?

Complete the neurological examination. If there is a complaint of a marked change in smell or taste, especially in a patient for whom it has more serious implications (a chef or a sommelier for example), this should be clearly documented in the medical records.

> **Clinical insight**
>
> Impaired function of the olfactory nerve is usually noticed as a change in how food tastes as well as how it smells.

3.6 The eyes: part 1 (CN II and III) – pupils, acuity, fields and fundi

Fundoscopy is a vital skill that is fundamental to the assessment of the neurological patient. Proficiency is only obtained with much practice: persevere! It affords direct visual inspection of the patient's vasculature and nervous system and, as such, is a uniquely informative bedside technique. There are virtually no systemic diseases that cannot affect the eye, and so being confident in fundoscopy is a benefit to those in all specialties.

Objective

The objective is to assess the optic nerve and the parasympathetic function of the oculomotor nerve.

Approach

Carry out this part of the assessment in a darkened room if possible. Inform the patient that they will have a bright light shone into their eyes, which they may find uncomfortable. Ask the patient to fixate on a distant object just above their head height. Dilate the pupils if required.

> **Guiding principle**
>
> Avoid the temptation to rush fundoscopy and pupillary responses and move onto eye movements. It is worth performing this stage properly as it allows assessment of the optic nerve, midbrain, thalamus (lateral geniculate nucleus), internal capsule, and parietal, temporal and occipital lobes and can be very helpful in localising pathology.

Equipment

An ophthalmoscope, pen torch, Snellen chart, hat pin, Ishihara plates and mydriatic drops are required.

Sequence

Pupils

To assess the pupils:

1. note the resting size, shape and symmetry of the pupils in both dim and bright light
2. elicit the pupillary reflex in each eye in turn
3. test the accommodation reaction. Ask the patient to fixate on your finger held a few feet in front of their face. Move your finger towards their nose and observe their pupils
4. test for a RAPD: shine a light in one eye and observe the other. Then, move the light to the eye being observed and note whether it elicits the same or less constriction. Repeat on the other eye.

Acuity

To assess the acuity:

1. use a Snellen chart. Normal acuity is '6/6' (metres) or '20/20' feet. '6/12' vision would represent the ability to read at

6 metres what can usually be read at 12 metres, i.e. reduced acuity

2. if the patient is unable to read the largest lettering on the chart, test if they can: (a) see the number of fingers you are holding up; (b) see hand movement; or (c) perceive light.

Colour vision

Colour vision can be abnormal before acuity and should also be tested with Ishihara plates if there are any concerns about vision.

Fields

Accurate assessment of any visual field loss helps to localise a lesion along the optic pathway. Lesions at particular sites along the pathway produce characteristic patterns of visual loss.

To assess the fields:

1. position your head in front of the patient's and at the same level. Ask them to close or cover one eye and close your own eye opposite

> ## Clinical insight
>
> A relative afferent pupillary defect is when a pupil appears to dilate in response to moving a light from the other eye onto it. It is caused by any damage to the retina or optic nerve on the affected side. This results in the observation that when a light is shone in the other, unaffected, eye the strong bilateral effector arm of the pupillary response causes a contralateral constriction of the other pupil. This is normal.
>
> When there is damage to the retina or optic disc, moving the light onto the affected eye will result in less stimulation of the afferent limb of the reflex and the pupil will dilate compared with when the light is in the other eye.

2. move a red hat pin into the field of vision from outside of it, asking the patient to say when they see the hat pin as red

3. repeat this in each of four quadrants for each eye, comparing the patient's field of vision with your own

4. assess the size of their blind spot

5. it is also convenient to test for visual neglect or extinction at this stage.

Blind spot

To assess the blind spot:

1. ask the patient to close one eye in turn

2. using the hat pin, find your own blind spot by holding it on the horizontal midline and moving the pin slowly laterally until the bright head of the pin disappears
3. if the examiner and patient's heads are at the same level the blind spots should be around the same spot
4. ask the patient to say when the pinhead disappears and reappears
5. map out any enlarged blind spot or scotoma

Visual neglect

To test for visual neglect, for each eye in turn:

- hold up a finger with each hand in two opposites of the visual quadrants
- wiggle the left, then the right, then both fingers and ask the patient to identify which moves

- in visual neglect the patient will fail to detect the movement on the affected side
- in visual extinction the movement will be initially detected when the finger is moved on its own but then failed to be appreciated when both fingers are moved simultaneously

> ### Clinical insight
>
> A common mistake in assessing fields and blind spots is to fail to present the hat pin midway between the examiner and the patient, thereby testing different visual fields of each party. Ensure you test midway by standing two arm's lengths back from the patient and presenting the hat pin at arm's length.

Fundoscopy

To examine the patient's fundi, ask them to remain fixated on a distant point:

1. using the ophthalmoscope light, check the red reflex in both eyes from a distance
2. use your right eye to examine the patient's right eye and your left eye to examine the patient's left eye
3. with your eye at the same level as the patient's, approach from about 20° laterally with one hand on their head with your thumb on the bony orbital margin of the eye you are examining

4. approach their eye until the retina comes into focus. You may need to get your head close enough that the ophthalmoscope touches your finger on the patient's orbit
5. identify an artery or vein and follow it back to the optic disc
6. examine the margins of the disc, checking that they are well defined and that there is no swelling or cupping and note its colour (an indistinct nasal margin is common)
7. examine the rest of the retina, taking each quadrant in turn and specifically looking for features of diabetic or hypertensive changes or any pigmentation
8. also note any signs of retinal detachment or artery or venous occlusion or thrombosis

Ophthalmoscope adjustment

The retina should come into focus with the lens set at 0 and the optic disc at red 2. Black is positive and focuses nearer; red is negative and focuses more distant.

Removing spectacles for fundoscopy is preferred as it allows closer examination but requires correction with the ophthalmoscope. Determine whether the patient is short or long sighted and adjust the ophthalmoscope accordingly. If the examiner also has a refractive error, it will either exaggerate the correction required, if it is the same type of error as the patient, or partially correct it, if it is the opposite. An approximate guide is to start with the lens at +8, visualise the lens and anterior chamber of the eye, and then move the lens down to 0 or below to bring the fundus into focus.

Key differential diagnoses
Pupils

If the pupils are unequal, determine whether one or both is inappropriately large or inappropriately small.

Large pupils (mydriasis)

The causes of a large pupil include:
- overactivity of the sympathetic system: some drugs of abuse (especially those with serotonergic properties such as ecstasy, cocaine and amphetamines)

- underactivity of the parasympathetic system: drugs (e.g. anticholinergics); trauma to CN III (including aneurysm of the posterior communicating aneurysm); Holmes–Adie syndrome (damage to postganglionic fibres from viral or bacterial infection resulting in mydriasis, areflexia and hyperhidrosis). A Holmes–Adie pupil should slowly constrict to accommodation

Small pupils (miosis)

The causes of a small pupil include:
- underactivity of the sympathetic system: e.g. Horner's syndrome of ptosis, miosis, anhidrosis and enophthalmos
- drugs: e.g. opioids, cholinergics, antipsychotics and organophosphates
- pontine lesions
- senile miosis

Light–near dissociation

This occurs when a pupil reacts to either light or accommodation but not both. There are a number of causes:
- a large pupil unreactive to light but that slowly accommodates is a Holmes–Adie pupil
- a small pupil unreactive to light but that accommodates is an Argyll Robertson pupil (a sign of tertiary syphilis)
- tonic pupils are similar to Argyll Robertson pupils except they are more common and accommodation is much slower and not associated with syphilis

Relative afferent pupillary defect

The causes include any unilateral retinal disorder such as ischaemic optic neuropathy, or unilateral optic neuritis, a common finding in multiple sclerosis even in the absence of overt optic neuritis.

Acuity

Rapid monocular visual loss

The causes include:
- retinal artery or vein occlusion
- ischaemic optic neuropathy
- optic neuritis
- giant cell arteritis
- migraine

Rapid binocular visual loss

The causes include:

- bilateral occipital lobe lesions (infarction, haemorrhage or trauma)
- bilateral optic neuritis or papillitis (infection, inflammation or infiltration)
- alcohol poisoning
- functional

Visual field defects

Concentric reduction of visual fields

This can be caused by retinal disease (such as retinitis pigmentosa), migraine or, if of gradual onset, papilloedema.

Central scotoma or enlarged blind spot

The causes of a central scotoma include optic nerve inflammation or demyelination, toxins or vascular disease.

Unilateral total visual field loss

Total loss of sight in one eye suggests an optic nerve or retinal lesion.

Bitemporal hemianopia

This is temporal visual field loss on each side, and can be caused by an optic chiasm lesion (e.g. pituitary tumour).

Homonymous hemianopia

This is where corresponding halves of the field are lost on each side. Any lesion from behind the optic chiasm to the occipital cortex, e.g. cortical stroke, can cause this. If there is macular sparing (i.e. the patient can read or see a hat pin in the midline) it suggests an incomplete occipital cortex lesion as this area is supplied by more than one vessel. If there is no macular sparing, it suggests a lesion in the optic radiation.

Homonymous quadrantanopia

If the visual field loss is in corresponding upper quadrants in both eyes, this indicates a lesion in optic radiation in the temporal lobe. If the visual field loss is in a lower quadrant, this indicates a lesion in optic radiation in the parietal lobe.

Fundi

Optic disc

The optic disc can appear swollen with a loss of normal shallow cup and clear rim and blurring of margins or pale:

- bilaterally swollen is most likely papilloedema
- unilateral swelling can be due to optic neuritis or papillitis
- pale with normal margins, caused by optic atrophy from, for example, optic neuritis
- pale with deep margins in glaucoma

Clinical insight

Clinically, papilloedema usually does not have severe visual loss until later on, whereas papillitis presents with early and severe loss of visual acuity.

Blood vessels

Look for arteriosclerotic and diabetic changes:

- arteriosclerotic changes: arteriolar narrowing, arteriovenous nipping (veins narrow as arteries cross them), silver wiring, flame haemorrhages (bleeding into the nerve fibre layer) and exudates
- diabetic changes: macular oedema, neovascularisation, cotton wool spots (retinal infarcts) and flame or dot–blot haemorrhages (**Table 3.6**)

What happens next?

After carrying out the sequences listed above:

- the neurological and general examination should be completed
- change in acuity should be recorded and investigated promptly
- any detected visual field loss should be formally mapped using automated perimetry
- brain imaging should be carried out if there is loss of acuity or visual field
- findings from fundoscopy should be investigated appropriately: treatment of hypertension; referral to ophthalmologists

for surveillance or treatment of diabetic retinopathy; brain imaging and lumbar puncture for papilloedema or optic neuritis

3.7 The eyes: part 2 (CN III, IV and VI)

Objective

The objective is to assess the integrity of control of eye movements. This is mainly focused on testing the motor functions of CN III, IV and VI (**Table 3.9**), including the whole neuroaxis from muscle to cortical centres.

Approach

There are three main types of eye movements: pursuit, saccadic and vestibulo-ocular:

- the occipital lobes direct control of pursuit (the slow eye movements used to track objects)
- the frontal lobes direct saccadic eye movements (the rapid movements from points of fixation)
- the cerebellar vestibular nuclei control the vestibulo-ocular movements (which maintain fixation during head movements)

Ensure that you are directly in front of the patient at eye level and that you give clear instructions and ask them to report the development of any double vision.

Muscle	Nerve	Primary action
Superior rectus	III	Elevation in abduction
Inferior rectus	III	Depression in abduction
Medial rectus	III	Adduction
Inferior oblique	III	Elevation in adduction
Lateral rectus	VI	Abduction
Superior oblique	IV	Depression in adduction

Table 3.9 The muscles and nerves of eye movements

Adduction will be normal with convergence as this does not involve the MLF (Figure 3.13).

Clinical insight

Distinguishing between a central and peripheral CN VII lesion is clinically very important as ischaemic central lesions are common causes of the former, and Bell's palsy is a common peripheral cause.

Key differential diagnoses

These are summarised in **Table 3.11**.

Any eye movement abnormality indicates MRIm, which provides higher resolution imaging of the brainstem and posterior fossa than a CT scan. Consider neuro-ophthalmological referral.

3.8 The face (CN V, VII)

Objective

The purpose of this part of the examination is to assess the functions of cranial nerves V and VII. CN V is largely sensory and parasympathetic but with some minor motor function. CN VII is largely motor but with sensory and parasympathetic function too.

Approach

Inform the patient that you will gently touch the very corner of their eye with a tiny piece of cotton wool. This is usually uncomfortable for them. Check whether they are wearing contact lenses before doing so.

Equipment

This requires a cotton wool swab, a Neurotip, tuning fork, universal containers with warm and cold water and a tendon hammer.

Sequence

Inspect for:

Lesion	Features	Causes
Generalised muscle or neuromuscular junction	Bilateral Multiple muscles Eyelids and facial muscle involvement Variable weakness Fatigability in myasthenia gravis (weakness worsens with repetition)	Myopathy Myasthenia gravis Lambert–Eaton myasthenic syndrome Myotonic dystrophy
Third nerve palsy	Eye 'down-and-out' (unopposed lateral rectus and superior oblique action) Ptosis Dilated unreactive pupil with preserved consensual reaction	Aneurysm Tumour Orbital lesion/mass, trauma Diabetes Migraine Basilar infarction (midbrain)
Fourth nerve palsy	Head tilt away from the side of the lesion Impaired depression in adduction Impaired intorsion of eye	Idiopathic Trauma Raised intracranial pressure Pontine infarction
Sixth nerve palsy	Impaired abduction Convergent strabismus	Idiopathic Trauma Raised intracranial pressure Basilar infarction
Conjugate gaze abnormalities	Internuclear ophthalmoplegia Supranuclear palsy	Lesion in MLF from multiple sclerosis or brainstem infarction Impaired voluntary vertical movements found in PSP and lesions in the dorsal midbrain
Skew deviation	One eye held higher than other Vertical diplopia	Midbrain or posterior fossa lesion, usually infarction
Opsoclonus	Rapid, involuntary, multidirectional saccadic movements	Midbrain lesion Idiopathic or tumour in children Inflammatory or paraneoplastic in adults
Macrosaccadic oscillations	Large saccadic movements overshooting target	Cerebellar lesions

Table 3.11 Key eye movement disorders and differential diagnoses. MLF, medial longitudinal fasciculus. PSP, progressive supranuclear palsy

1. wasting of the masseter or temporalis muscles
2. flattening of the nasolabial folds
3. presence of forehead wrinkles
4. spontaneous blinking or facial expressions
5. parotid gland swelling

CN V

After carrying out the initial inspection (above), assess CN V as follows.

Assess sensory component

Three main divisions each supply a different portion of the head: the ophthalmic division, the maxillary nerve and the mandibular nerve. Test each in turn on both sides:

1. use an examination pin (be gentle!) or the end of a clean paperclip (if no examination pins are available) to assess pain perception
2. other modalities are difficult to test as vibration tends to be felt diffusely and proprioception is not really possible! Use a universal container with warm and one with cold water to test temperature if needed
3. touch the tip to the forehead (V_1) on each side, asking the patient whether it feels sharp and to compare the sensation on both sides. Repeat just lateral to the cheekbones (V_2) and then either side of the chin (V_3)
4. if an area of altered sensation is detected map it out in more detail. Remember that the C2 dermatome begins near the back of the head and the area below the angle of the jaw is also C2/3 and should be normal in lesions of the trigeminal nerve

Assess motor function

To do this:

1. ask the patient to clench their teeth and feel the jaw for muscle bulk
2. ask them to keep their mouth open while you attempt to shut it. In unilateral lesions the jaw will deviate towards the weak side

3. test the jaw jerk. Ask the patient to loosely open their mouth and place the tip of your finger gently on their chin. Tap your finger softly with a tendon hammer to elicit any jaw jerk.

CN VII

Both motor and sensory functions of the facial nerve need to be assessed.

CN VII motor function

Ask the patient to:
1. lift their eyebrows (frontalis muscle)
2. screw their eyes tight shut (orbicularis oculi)
3. smile, then show their teeth
4. puff their cheeks and then whistle (buccinator and orbicularis oris)
5. demonstrate the movements if the patient fails to understand
6. observe for any asymmetry and test the strength of the movements with gentle pressure when possible
7. ask the patient whether they have become more sensitive to loud noises, which may indicate the hyperacusis of stapedius muscle weakness

CN VII sensory function (chorda tympani branch) – taste

Ask the patient:
1. whether they have had any change in their sense of taste. This is usually sufficient. It can be more formally assessed using drops of sugar, vinegar and salt on each side of the anterior two-thirds of the tongue in turn

> ## Clinical insight
>
> Bell's phenomenon is a normal phenomenon in which closure of the eyelid results in upward movement of the eyeball. It can be seen if one holds a patient's eyelid open and asks them to attempt to close their eyes. In patients with a CN VII nerve palsy that results in impaired eyelid closure, asking the patient to close their eyes will result in Bell's phenomenon being apparent without having to hold the eyelid open.

2. whether they have dry eyes. The greater petrosal nerve supplies parasympathetic activity to the lacrimal glands

(among other functions). Damage to the facial nerve may cause a decrease in tear production

Corneal reflex (CN V and VII)

Finally, test the corneal reflex with a fine wisp of cotton wool:

1. ask the patient to look up and to the right. Dab the wool into the lower corner of their left eye, being careful not to touch the conjunctivae. Repeat on the right, having asked them to look up and to the left
2. the afferent limb is carried by the ophthalmic division of the trigeminal nerve, and the efferent by the facial nerve innervation of orbicularis oculi
3. the reflex is consensual, meaning that if it is triggered on one side it should occur on both
4. palpate the parotid glands for any masses because these can cause damage to the facial nerve as it passes through it

People used to wearing contact lenses may have a reduced or absent corneal reflex. **Figure 3.14** illustrates the effects of a CN V and CN VII lesion on the corneal reflex.

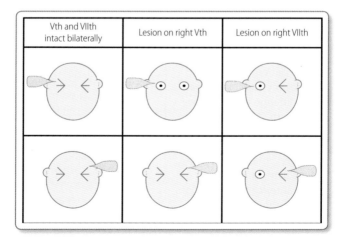

Vth and VIIth intact bilaterally	Lesion on right Vth	Lesion on right VIIth

Figure 3.14 The corneal reflex.

CN V motor lesion

CN V motor lesions cause:

- wasting or weakness: muscle disease such as myotonic dystrophy, some muscular dystrophies, motor neuron disease
- positive jaw jerk: indicates an UMN lesion; causes include stroke or motor neuron disease

CN V sensory lesion

Figure 3.5 shows likely lesion locations to account for common types of CN V sensory loss.

CN VII motor lesion

Upper motor neuron lesions

(e.g. stroke) These will often 'spare the forehead' because the LMNs of the facial nerve to frontalis (and sometimes orbicularis oculi) which originate in the pons receive UMN input from both the ipsilateral and contralateral motor cortices. Sometimes, a very subtle droop of the mouth is all that is apparent.

Lower motor neuron lesions

(e.g. Bell's palsy) These will often be fairly dramatic with full involvement of all the muscles, including frontalis and orbicularis oculi, because the lesion is at the final point of input to the muscle (i.e. the innervating motor neurons).

Bilateral lesions

These may represent muscle disease rather than nerve involvement, or be caused by Guillain–Barré syndrome, sarcoidosis, Lyme disease or tuberculosis, although these are all rare conditions. Other causes include tumours (including parotid tumours), syrinx and multiple sclerosis. Trigeminal neuralgia will cause paroxysms of intense electric shock-like pain in the distribution of the trigeminal nerve.

What happens next?

Obvious Bell's palsy or typical trigeminal neuralgia may not need brain imaging. Most lesions involving the trigeminal or facial nerves will require MRI of the posterior fossa and brainstem. Acute lesions should be assumed to be brainstem or cortical infarctions and investigated promptly.

3.9 The ears (CN VIII)

Objective
The objective is to assess the auditory and vestibular functions of the vestibulocochlear nerve.

Approach
Vestibular assessment is indicated if there are symptoms suggestive of vertigo, dizziness, nystagmus, posterior circulation involvement or a cerebellopontine angle lesion. Gross auditory dysfunction may be evident from the history taking. Specific symptoms or other findings may indicate more detailed testing if a lesion is suspected.

Equipment
This part of the examination requires an otoscope and a 512-Hz tuning fork.

Sequence
To test the auditory nerve:
1. inspect the head and external ear for any scars, hearing devices or local lymphadenopathy
2. inspect the internal auditory canal with the otoscope
3. visualise the tympanic membrane, which should be concave, free from excessive wax and with a light reflex on the anterior–inferior portion. Note any exudate or growth such as a cholesteotoma
4. cover one ear and whisper a number in the other from about 60 cm away. Repeat on the other side
5. Rinne's test and Weber's test should be performed if there are any reported symptoms or signs of hearing loss

Rinne's test
Rinne's test is performed as follows (**Figure 3.15**):
1. place the tuning fork on the mastoid process
2. when the patient cannot hear it, move it in front of the ear on the same side
3. ask if they can hear the tone

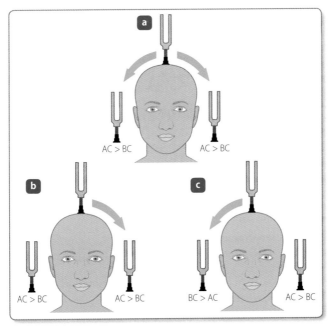

AC > BC   AC > BC

AC > BC   AC > BC

BC > AC   AC > BC

Figure 3.15 Rinne's and Weber's tests: (a) normal hearing: Weber's test is heard centrally; Rinne's test is positive on both sides, with air conduction greater than bone conduction. (b) Sensorineural deafness in the right ear: Weber's test lateralises to the better hearing (left) side; Rinne's test is positive on both sides. (c) Conductive deafness in the right ear: Weber's test lateralises to the affected right ear; Rinne's test is negative on the right side (bone conduction > air conduction) and positive on the normal left side (air conduction > bone conduction).

4. vibration on the mastoid tests bone conduction
5. air conduction is tested when the tuning fork is in front of the ear

Normally, the tone should be heard when the tuning fork is moved in front of the ear (Rinne positive):

- with sensorineural hearing loss air conduction remains better than bone conduction
- with conductive loss the tone is not heard in front of the ear (Rinne negative)

Weber's test

Weber's test is performed as follows (**Figure 3.15**):

1. place the tuning fork on the centre of the patient's forehead
2. ask if they hear it more in one ear
3. normally it is heard equally in both ears
4. with sensorineural loss, the tone is heard better in the unaffected ear
5. with conduction loss, the tone is better heard in the affected ear

The vestibular nerve

Next, assess the vestibular nerve. This should include assessment of gait (see Chapter 2), nystagmus (see Chapter 6) and bedside tests of vestibular function: Hallpike's test and the head turning test.

Hallpike's manoeuvre

This is a test to induce vertigo and confirm benign paroxysmal positional vertigo (BPPV):

1. ask the patient to sit on the bed so that their body and head can be lowered backwards over the edge
2. turn their head to one side
3. lower their head backwards over the edge
4. ask them to keep their eyes open and to look at your eyes. Observe for any nystagmus. The onset of this may be delayed so wait at least 30 seconds

Note any delay, the nature and direction of the nystagmus and whether the it fatigues with repetition of the test. Rapid onset and persistent nystagmus indicates a central vestibular lesion, whereas a peripheral lesion is indicated by fatigable nystagmus with a delayed onset.

Unterberger test

This tests for a vestibular lesion. Ask the patient to stand with their eyes closed and arms stretched out in front of the them and march on the spot. Note whether they turn to one side on the spot. This indicates a vestibular lesion on that side.

Key differential diagnoses

Deafness: sensorineural

There are a wide range of causes, including noise; presbycusis, otosclerosis, Ménière's disease, tumours at the cerebellopontine angle (e.g. acoustic neuroma), trauma, toxins, and infarction or demyelination of the brainstem or nerve fibre.

Deafness: conductive

Common causes of conductive deafness include wax, otitis media and other middle ear disease.

Vestibular lesion

Important causes include labyrinthitis; toxins; vestibular neuronitis; infarction or demyelination of nuclei or nerve; and tumour at the cerebellopontine angle.

What happens next?

Formal hearing tests should be arranged for acute or progressive hearing loss not readily attributed to noise exposure or presbycusis. Suspicion of a posterior fossa lesion will require MRI, including high resolution imaging for a suspected cerebellopontine angle tumour.

The Epley manoeuvre

BPPV can be treated at the bedside with repeated cycles of the Epley manoeuvre, a technique to reposition the misplaced otoconia from the semicircular canals to the utricle:

1. lie the patient flat on their back
2. turn the patient's head to the symptomatic side (this will have been the side lower down during a positive Hallpike's test)
3. wait 1 minute
4. turn the patient's head to face the ceiling for 1 minute
5. turn their head and body to face the direction opposite to the first for 1 minute
6. sit the patient up

3.10 The mouth (CN IX, X, XII)

For convenience, the lower cranial nerves are not all tested in order; rather, specific instructions are given that test key parts of various nerves.

Objective

The purpose of this part of the examination is to assess the function of the lower cranial nerves. The IXth, Xth and XIIth cranial nerves have similar origins, intracranial and initial extracranial courses, and are commonly affected together.

Approach

Inform the patient that you will need to look in their mouth, press down on their tongue and touch the back of their throat and that they may find this uncomfortable.

Equipment

To carry out this part of the examination, a tongue depressor, 'orange stick' or throat swab, and pen torch are required.

Sequence

Carry out the following steps in turn:
1. ask the patient to open their mouth; inspect the palate and tongue using a pen torch
2. note the position of the uvula and whether there is any deviation (CN X)
3. look for fasciculations or wasting of the tongue (CN XII)
4. ask the patient to say 'Ah' and watch for elevation of the uvula (CN X). This should be central. Unilateral lesions of the vagus nerve will draw the uvula to the normal side and bilateral lesions will result in no movement
5. ask them to protrude their tongue straight out (it will deviate to the weak side) and then to move it back and forth; note any stiffness or slowness (CN XII)
6. ask the patient to speak, noting any dysarthria (CN IX, X or XII) or hoarseness (CN X)
7. have them cough (CN X) and swallow some water (CN IX, X and XII)

8. test the gag reflex using the tongue depressor and the throat swab. Touch the back of the pharynx on each side, observing for a contraction of the soft palate. Ask the patient if they felt the touch on each side
9. taste on the posterior third of the tongue can be tested to examine the function of the CN IXth nerve; however, unless an isolated CN IX lesion is suspected it is not commonly performed

Key differential diagnoses

The IXth and Xth nerves are commonly affected together or with the XIth and XIIth nerves as syndromes (**Table 3.4**). It is useful to describe the findings and determine whether there is a central or peripheral cause.

Findings

Common findings are:

- dysarthria
- dysphonia
- deviated uvula
- abnormal gag reflex
- poor cough

Central

Important central nervous system causes include:

- lateral medullary infarction
- syrinx
- tumours
- motor neuron disease

Peripheral

Important peripheral causes include:

- tumours (e.g. metastasis at the jugular foramen)
- aneurysms

> ## Clinical insight
>
> Autonomic functions of CN IX and X:
>
> The carotid reflex is central to blood pressure homeostasis. CN IX mediates the afferent limb from baroreceptors monitoring blood pressure in the carotid bodies and carotid sinus, whereas many efferent responses are mediated via the vagus. It is difficult to detect subtle dysfunction clinically but the carotid reflex can be assessed by an ECG recording of heart rate (HR):
>
> - respiration: HR should vary <10 bpm at rest
> - standing: HR should increase by >10 bpm
> - Valsalva manoeuvre: increase in HR
> - carotid massage: decrease in HR
> - lying and standing blood pressure should differ by no more than 30 mmHg systolic or 15 mmHg diastolic

- basal meningitis
- peripheral nerve disorders (e.g. Guillain–Barré syndrome)
- glossopharyngeal neuralgia
- mediastinal pathology can involve the vagus nerve

What happens next?

Patients with lower cranial nerve lesions should have a formal assessment by qualified speech and language therapists and an otolaryngologist to determine the nature and extent of their speech and swallow disturbances. Imaging of the posterior fossa, base of the skull and neck is indicated. Electromyography (EMG) is indicated if motor neuron disease is suspected.

3.11 The neck (CN XI)

Objective

This part of the examination assesses the function of the accessory nerve (XI).

Approach

CN XI is a purely motor nerve that innervates the sternocleido-mastoid and trapezius muscles. General inspection of the neck is appropriate at this stage and palpation for lymphadenopathy should also be performed.

Sequence

Inspect the neck, looking for:
- head drop suggestive of muscle disease/dystrophy
- fasciculations or wasting of sternocleidomastoid or trapezius
- any scars or swellings

Following the inspection:
1. ask the patient to shrug their shoulders. Push down on them to assess strength
2. ask them to turn their head to the right and then attempt to straighten it. This tests the left sternocleidomastoid muscle. Repeat for the other side
3. palpate for any lymphadenopathy

Key differential diagnoses

Isolated CN XI lesions are rare. More commonly, CN XI is affected as part of a cranial nerve syndrome (**Table 3.4**). Causes are classified as central or peripheral, or relating to any observed lymphadenopathy.

Central

These include:
- medullary infarction
- syrinx
- motor neuron disease
- high cervical injury

Peripheral

These include:
- neck trauma, including surgery
- muscle disorders/dystrophies
- peripheral neuropathies
- motor neuron disease

Lymphadenopathy

This includes the following:
- any cause of cervical lymphadenopathy
- lymph nodes may directly compress the accessory nerve
- lymphadenopathy in the context of neurological dysfunction may indicate a paraneoplastic syndrome

What happens next?

Spinal cord and brain imaging is indicated in lesions of CN XI. Nerve conduction or EMG is also helpful. Lymphadenopathy should be investigated in the usual manner. In the context of suspected paraneoplastic syndromes this should include biopsy; a breast examination and gynaecological assessment in women; a testicular examination in men; a chest radiograph; and usually CT of the chest, abdomen and pelvis and consideration of a positron emission tomography (PET) scan.

3.12 System summary

A summary of cranial nerve examination is given in **Table 3.12**.

General inspection	Syndromes Generalised neurological disease Generalised non-neurological disease
CN I: the nose	Ask about smell and taste
CN II and III: the eyes 1	Pupils Acuity Fields Fundi
CN III, IV and VI: the eyes 2	Resting position Cover test Pursuits Saccades
CN V and VII: the face	Facial sensation Muscles of mastication Jaw jerk Muscles of facial expression Hyperacusis Taste Lacrimation Corneal reflex Palpate parotids
CN VIII: the ears	Otoscopy Whisper Rinne's and Weber's tests Gait Nystagmus Hallpike's and head turning test
CN IX, X and XII: the mouth	Uvula Tongue Voice Cough Swallow Gag reflex
CN XI: the neck	Sternocleidomastoid Trapezius Lymphadenopathy

Table 3.12 Summary of cranial nerve examination

Upper limb

4.1 Objectives

Examination of the upper limb aims to further identify any neurological deficit, localise it and aid in determining the underlying pathological process.

There is a traditional routine that neurologists follow:
- general inspection
- tone
- power
- reflexes
- co-ordination
- sensation

Think: **To** (tone) **Postpone** (power) **Reflexes** (reflexes) **Constitutes** (co-ordination) **Sacrilege** (sensation).

There are three aims of this stage of the examination:
1. identify any syndrome or obvious abnormalities from general inspection
2. determine whether there is an upper motor neuron (UMN) or lower motor neuron (LMN) lesion
3. determine whether the lesion is cortical, spinal, root, peripheral nerve or muscle

Students most often get lost at step 3, but some sound anatomy and a systematic examination routine are all that is required.

4.2 Anatomy and physiology review

Table 4.1 summarises the major functions of the main nerves of the upper limb. All the major nerves of the upper limb have both a motor and a sensory component. **Figure 4.1** shows the dermatomes.

Upper and lower motor neurons

The motor system comprises UMNs and LMNs (**Figure 4.2**). The LMN is the α-motor neuron in the anterior horn of the spinal

Nerve	Root	Cord of plexus	Sensory	Key muscles	Muscle action
Axillary	C5/6	Posterior	Patch on shoulder	Deltoid	Abducts arm
Radial	C6/7	Posterior	Dorsolateral arm and forearm	Triceps Extensor digitorum Abductor pollicis longus	Extends elbow Extends fingers Abducts thumb
Musculocutaneous	C5/6	Lateral	Lateral forearm	Biceps	Flexes elbow
Median	C8/T1	Lateral and medial	Lateral 2/3 of the palm and 3½ digits	Pronator teres Flexor carpi radialis Flexor pollicis longus Opponens pollicis Flexor digitorum profundus I and II	Pronates forearm Flexes and abducts wrist Flexes distal phalanx of thumb Opposes thumb Flexes distal phalanx of index and middle fingers
Ulnar	C8/T1	Medial	Medial 1/3 of the palm and dorsum of the hand. Little finger and medial ½ ring finger	Flexor carpi ulnaris 1st dorsal interosseous 2nd palmar interosseous Adductor pollicis Flexor digitorum profundus III and IV	Abducts little finger Abducts index finger Adducts index finger Adducts thumb Flexes distal phalanx of ring and little fingers

Table 4.1 Summary of the main upper limb peripheral nerve origins and functions

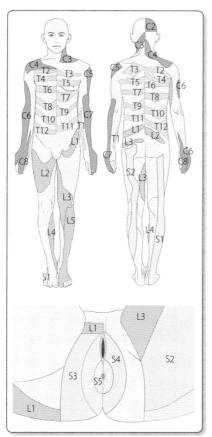

Figure 4.1 Sensory dermatomes.

cord which innervates the muscle fibre. The UMN is the cell or cells directly involved in supplying input to the LMN (e.g. the pyramidal cells in layer V of the motor cortex).

The LMN is the final output pathway to the muscle. Thus if its cell body in the spinal cord or brainstem, or if the nerve root or peripheral nerve is damaged there is no other way for

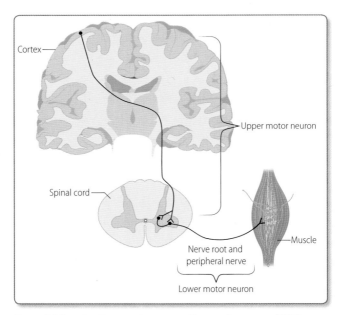

Figure 4.2 Upper and lower motor neurons. Upper motor neurons (UMN) originate in the motor cortex and descend to the brainstem or spinal cord where they synapse on interneurons and the cell bodies of lower motor neurons (LMN). LMN cell bodies originate in the brainstem or spinal cord, and send their axons out via the cranial or peripheral nerves to target muscles.

the muscle to be activated and it loses its tonic activation and trophic support. The muscle then becomes flaccid, it wastes and the reflex arc is broken.

The UMN is part of a more complex afferent supply to the LMN. Damage to the UMNs, in the spinal cord, brainstem, cerebellum or cortex, leads to increased tonic activation of the unaffected α-motor neuron (probably through local disinhibition in the spinal cord), which remains intact and capable of muscle activation. The muscle becomes spastic and very sensitive to reflex stimulation. It is however weak and may atrophy with time through disuse.

Musculocutaneous nerve

Key anatomy of the musculocutaneous nerve:

- roots C5/6
- lateral cord of the brachial plexus
- sensory: lateral cutaneous nerve of the forearm (lateral forearm from the elbow to the wrist)
- motor: biceps brachii (flexes supinated forearm), brachialis (synergist to biceps)

Axillary nerve

Key anatomy of the axillary nerve:

- roots C5/6
- posterior cord of the brachial plexus
- sensory: patch on the lateral aspect of the shoulder
- motor: deltoid (abducts the upper arm)

Radial nerve

Key anatomy of the radial nerve:

- divides after the antecubital fossa to give the posterior interosseous nerve (PIN) and superficial radial nerve
- roots C5–8 (mostly C6/7)
- posterior cord of the brachial plexus
- sensory: posterior cutaneous nerve of the arm (dorsolateral aspect of the upper arm), posterior cutaneous nerve of the forearm (dorsolateral surface of the hand)
- motor: extensor muscles of the upper limb. Key muscles include: triceps (radial; extends forearm, C7), extensor carpi radialis longus (radial; extends and abducts the hand at the wrist, C6), extensor carpi ulnaris (PIN; extends and adducts the hand at the wrist, C7), extensor digitorum (PIN; extension of the fingers at the metacarpophalangeal joints, C7), abductor pollicis longus (PIN; abducts the thumb at the carpometacarpal joint, C7)

Clinical insight

Radial nerve palsy results in:

- wrist drop
- weakness of thumb extension
- numbness over the dorsolateral aspect of the hand

Causes include compression in the axilla, humeral fracture or compression from supinator.

Median nerve

Key anatomy of the median nerve:

- anterior interosseous nerve (AIN) branches off after the antecubital fossa. The palmar sensory branch divides before the carpal tunnel
- roots C6–T1 (mostly C8/T1)
- lateral and medial cords of the brachial plexus
- sensory: palmar sensory branch – the lateral aspect of the palm from the lateral half of the base of the ring finger to the proximal phalanx of the thumb; portion through carpal tunnel – palmar surface of the first, second and lateral half of the third fingers, dorsal aspect of the same and the distal phalanx of the thumb
- motor: all flexors in the forearm except flexor carpi ulnaris and part of flexor digitorum profundus. Key muscles include: pronator teres (median; pronates the forearm, C6/7), flexor carpi radialis (median; flexes and abducts the hand at the wrist, C6/7), flexor pollicis longus (AIN; flexes the distal phalanx of the thumb, C8), flexor digitorum profundus I and II (AIN; flexes the distal phalanx of the index and middle fingers, C8), abductor pollicis brevis (median; abducts the thumb at right angles to the palm, T1), opponens pollicis (median; opposes the thumb and little finger, T1), first and second lumbricals (median; extends the finger at the proximal interphalangeal joint, T1)

Clinical insight

LOAF is a useful mnemonic for the main motor functions of the median nerve:

L   first and second **L**umbricals

O   **O**pponens pollicis

A   **A**bductor pollicis brevis

F   **F**lexor pollicis longus

Clinical insight

Carpal tunnel syndrome (entrapment at the wrist):

- numbness or paraesthesias in the thumb, first and second fingers
- may progress to weakness in fine movements of the hands
- thenar muscles may atrophy

Median nerve entrapment (above the wrist):

- pain above the elbow or forearm
- weakness in pronation

Ulnar nerve

Key anatomy of the ulnar nerve:

- medial cutaneous nerves of the arm and forearm branch off at the proximal medial cord of the brachial plexus. Dorsal and palmar cutaneous braches leave in the forearm. Deep motor and superficial terminal branches enter the hand
- roots C8/T1
- medial cord of the brachial plexus
- sensory: little finger and medial half of the ring finger, and the palmar and dorsal aspects of the hand below the little finger and the medial half of the ring finger
- motor: 'ulnar flexing' and most of the small muscles of the hand. Key muscles include: flexor digitorum profundus III and IV (flexes the distal phalanx of the ring and little fingers, C8), flexor carpi ulnaris (abducts the little finger, C8), flexor digiti minimi (flexes the little finger at the metacarpophalangeal joint, T1), first dorsal interosseous (abducts the index finger, T1), second palmar interosseous (adducts the index finger, T1), adductor pollicis (adducts the thumb at right angles to the palm, T1)

Brachial plexus

The brachial plexus is a network of nerves formed from the cervical roots and T1 as they re-sort to form the peripheral nerves (**Figure 4.3**).

It is organised so that:

- five roots join to form three trunks (upper, middle, lower)

> ### Clinical insight
>
> Ulnar nerve palsy:
> - numbness or paraesthesia in the ring and little finger
> - weakness of finger abduction
> - symptoms worsened by elbow flexion
> - causes: compression in the ulnar groove, wrist or palm

- three trunks split/join to form three cords (lateral, posterior, medial)
- three cords split/join to form the five major peripheral nerves
- In addition to the muscles innervated by the major peripheral nerves ultimately formed from the trunks and cords, there are additional smaller nerves that branch off cords and trunks and aid in localisation

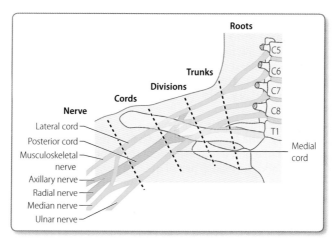

Figure 4.3 Brachial plexus.

Sensory function

The sensory function of the limbs is divided into four modalities:
1. pain [assessed by pin-prick testing (PP)]
4. temperature (T°C)
5. joint position sense (JPS)
6. vibration sense (Vib)

Pain and temperature fibres decussate in the spinal cord via the anterior commissure at the level they enter it and are carried in the contralateral lateral columns (**Figure 4.4**). JPS and Vib are carried in the ipsilateral dorsal columns and decussate at the level of the medulla. 'Light touch' is sensed via a combination of lateral and dorsal columns and is not a clinically useful examination method.

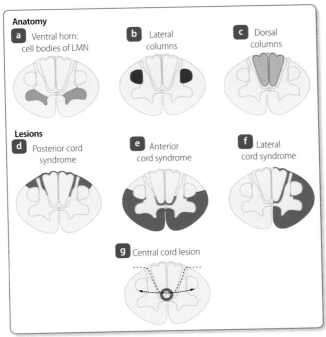

Figure 4.4 Spinal cord anatomy and lesions. (a) Ventral horn, showing cell bodies of lower motor neurons (green) (b) Lateral columns (purple) receive pinprick (PP) and temperature (T°C) sensation input from the contralateral body via fibres crossing the midline through the anterior commissure. (c) Dorsal columns (orange) receive joint position sense (JPS) and vibration sense (Vib) from the ipsilateral body via fibres that cross at the medulla. (d) Posterior cord syndrome. Loss of JPS and Vib below the lesion. (e) Anterior cord syndrome. Loss of PP and T°C sensation and weakness below the lesion. (f) Lateral cord syndrome. Loss of ipsilateral JPS and Vib and contralateral PP and T°C sensation and weakness below the lesion. (g) Central cord lesion: disruption of the crossing PP and T°C fibres supplying the lateral columns.

4.3 Clinical features and pathophysiology

General inspection

Assess patient for:

- **abnormal posture**: e.g. pyramidal distribution of weakness where there is greater weakness in the arm extensors than in the flexors leading to a flexed elbow and wrist. This indicates an UMN lesion, e.g. cortical stroke or mass lesion (e.g. tumour, abscess, haematoma)
- **wasting**: guttering of the interosseous muscles; flattening of the thenar or hypothenar eminences. This indicates a LMN lesion or chronic UMN lesion
- **fasciculations**: spontaneous single muscle fibre contractions appearing as rippling of muscles. These indicate denervation and re-innervation of the neuromuscular junction, usually from LMN lesions
- **pronator drift**: one arm will slowly pronate when the arms are in front and the eyes closed. This is quite a sensitive marker of an UMN lesion in the corticospinal tract
- **syndromic appearance**: remember the more common syndromes

Patterns of weakness

These include:

- **UMN lesion**: produces increased tone, hyper-reflexia and spastic weakness
- **LMN lesion**: produces reduced tone, low or absent reflexes and flaccid weakness
- **neuromuscular junction**: relatively rare, this will give characteristic fatigable weakness in myasthenia gravis (i.e. weakness gets worse on repetitive movements) or facilitation in Lambert–Eaton myasthenic syndrome (i.e. weakness improves after a few contractions). It tends to affect highly active muscles, including the extraocular muscles. Reflexes and sensation are normal
- **muscle**: similar to a LMN lesion with wasting, reduced tone and reflexes reduced in proportion to weakness. There is huge variation; distribution may be more proximal, with pain, cramps, spasms or muscle tenderness

- **functional**: weakness variable, 'non-anatomical', often muscles' give way' with an initially normal effort that suddenly fails, may have normal reflexes and sensory findings. 'Functional overlay' can complicate the clinical presentation of genuine or long-standing weakness

Patterns of sensory disturbance
Pain
Pain is usually mentioned in the history. Its nature can reflect its cause:

- **neuropathic pain** is usually described as sharp, stabbing, shooting, lancing, electric shocks, etc.
- **radicular pain** has the distribution of a dermatome
- **radiculopathy** is when there are also sensory signs or motor signs
- **small fibre** peripheral neuropathies can be painful in the typical nerve distribution or glove-and-stocking pattern
- **brachial plexitis** is a rare, probably autoimmune, condition in which there is acute shoulder pain followed by multifocal LMN weakness in the affected arm
- **central pain** describes a form of neuropathic pain presumed to come from lesions in the central nervous system (CNS), e.g. thalamic pain is a neuropathic-type pain in a hemi-sensory distribution secondary to lesions (usually infarcts) in the sensory thalamus

Paraesthesia
'Tingly bits' are a common complaint in the neurologist's clinic. The causes range from anxiety or functional disorders to peripheral nerve, root and spinal cord lesions. If they are the sole symptom and the examination is normal they are rarely - despite patient's fears – a presentation of central lesions such as tumours.

Patients may describe pins and needles, watery sensations, sharp sensations, tightness, burning, heaviness, etc. The distribution is often helpful:

- **glove and stocking** may be early peripheral neuropathy (progresses) or anxiety (fluctuates; may also be perioral during hyperventilation)

- typical **peripheral nerve distribution** in a peripheral nerve lesion
- **dermatomal** distribution, along with pain, indicates nerve root lesions or spinal cord lesions such as transverse myelitis or multiple sclerosis
- **hemi-sensory** distribution may represent a thalamic lesion or sensory cortical lesion or simple partial seizure or migraine
- **non-anatomical distribution** indicates functional disorders. The closer to a recognisable anatomical distribution the more a structural cause should be sought

Sensory loss

Careful attention to the pattern and modalities of sensory loss on examination can greatly aid localisation. Causes of sensory loss include:

- **peripheral nerve/plexus**: 'trapped nerves' give sensory loss in the whole nerve distribution below the lesion
- **polyneuropathies** are usually length dependent, meaning that the longer nerves (distal sensation) are affected first, leading to the classic glove-and-stocking distribution

> ### Clinical insight
>
> Severe polyneuropathies can look like a spinal cord lesion if the more proximal peripheral nerves are affected. A spinal cord lesion will give a spinal level where there is complete loss of affected modalities below the lesion, whereas even a severe polyneuropathy will usually spare a region of sensation in a strip running down the midline of the back.
>
> This is because the paraspinal cutaneous nerves are among the shortest nerves and last to be affected in a neuropathy. Therefore, when a spinal lesion is clinically suspected always check sensation down the spine itself to exclude a severe length-dependent polyneuropathy.

- **stroke** will typically cause sensory loss rather than positive phenomena such as pain or paraesthesia
- **nerve root**: sensory loss may be in only one or two modalities at first but is usually associated with radicular pain
- **dorsal column**: lesions here cause a loss of JPS and Vib sensation below and ipsilateral to the side of the lesion (contralateral if the lesion is above the decussation in the medulla). Patients may complain of ataxia or clumsiness

- **lateral column**: lesions here cause a loss of PP and T°C sensation below and contralateral to the side of the lesion. Patients may complain of injuring or burning their extremities

4.4 General observations

Objective
The objective of the general observations is to identify any neurological syndromes or obvious weakness, deformity, abnormal posture, wasting or fasciculations.

Approach
The patient undresses to their underwear to enable full assessment of their muscles and nerves. Instruct women to keep their bra on.

Sequence
In generally assessing the upper limb, observe from in front and then behind. Look for:
1. **asymmetry** in posture of the upper limbs, e.g. contracted spastic hemiplegia
7. **muscle wasting,** particularly the first dorsal interosseous and the thenar and hypothenar eminences
8. **fasciculations**: these may be evident only after prolonged observation
9. **pronator drift**: ask the patient to 'put your hands out in front of you, palms up, and close your eyes'

Key differential diagnoses
Key differentials include:
- abnormal posture of one arm: dystonia, simple partial seizure, hemiplegia
- muscle wasting: a LMN lesion causes denervation of muscle and atrophy. Long-standing UMN lesions can eventually cause wasting through disuse
- fasciculations: benign (e.g. young patient, after exercise), motor neuron disease, any cause of denervation (i.e. LMN lesion)
- pronator drift: corticospinal tract lesions will cause the affected limb to pronate and flex at the elbow

What happens next?
The next step is to examine tone.

4.5 Tone

Objective
The purpose of this part of the examination is to identify any pathologically increased or decreased tone.

Sequence
To assess the tone of the upper limb:
1. take the patients hand as though to shake it
2. tell them 'let me take the weight of your arm'
3. flex and extend and rotate the arm at the wrist, elbow and shoulder at variable speed
4. ask the patient to 'open and close your other fist' to accentuate any increased tone

Key differential diagnoses
These are as follows:
- **increased tone** indicates increased tonic activation of an intact LMN. Can also be normal or from anxiety
- **spasticity** is a velocity-dependent increase in tone (i.e. the arm becomes stiffer the faster it is moved) and indicates an UMN lesion
- spasticity with superimposed tremor occurs in parkinsonism. It is described as **'cog-wheeling'**
- **reduced tone** indicates decreased tonic activation of muscles. This generally indicates a LMN or muscle lesion
- **hyperacute UMN** lesions can sometimes cause flaccid weakness (e.g. an acute stroke)

What happens next?
The next step is to examine power.

4.6 Power

Objective
This stage is used to examine the strength of individual muscles and thereby indirectly peripheral nerve, brachial plexus, nerve root and CNS function.

Approach
The patient is asked to move their arms into various positions and then the examiner attempts to overcome their strength. **Table 4.2** shows how muscle strength is graded.

Sequence
The sequence tests the muscles in turn in a logical order to assess a number of muscles from each major peripheral nerve and nerve root. The verbal instructions are given in **Table 4.3**, as is the muscle being tested, the innervating nerve, the supplying brachial plexus cord and the major root. **Figures 4.5–4.8** demonstrate a useful order in which to test the key muscles.

Grade	Description
0	No movement
1	Perceptible flicker of muscle contraction
2	Movement only if gravity eliminated
3	Can overcome gravity but not resistance
4	Can be overcome by examiner
5	Normal strength

Table 4.2 Medical Research Council (MRC) power grade. Sometimes grade 4 is designated 4+ when there is considerable but not full strength, and designated 4- when easily overpowered

Instruction	Muscle	Muscle action	Nerve	Plexus cord	Root
Lift your elbows up and out	Deltoid	Shoulder abduction	Ax	P	C5/6
Make arms like a boxer	Biceps brachii	Elbow flexion	MS	L	C5/6
Make arms like a boxer	Triceps	Elbow extension	R	P	C7
Make fists and cock your wrists back	Extensor carpi radialis longus	Wrist extension and abduction	R	P	C6
Make fists and cock your wrists back	Extensor carpi ulnaris	Wrist extension and adduction	R	P	C7
Keep your fingers out straight	Extensor digitorum	Finger extension	R	P	C7
Stick your thumbs out to the side	Extensor pollicis brevis	Thumb abduction	R	P	C7
Grip my finger tips	Flexor digitorum profundus I and II	Flexion of distal phalanx	Md	L, MI	C8
Bend your thumbs	Flexor pollicis longus	Flexion of thumb	Md	L, MI	C8
Touch your thumbs to the base of your little finger	Opponens pollicis	Thumb opposition	Md	L, MI	T1
Spread your fingers wide	Flexor carpi ulnaris	Finger abduction	U	MI	C8
Spread your fingers wide	1st dorsal interosseous	Finger abduction	U	MI	T1
Keep your fingers together	2nd palmar interosseous	Finger adduction	U	MI	T1
Keep your thumb on your palm	Adductor pollicis	Thumb adduction	U	MI	T1

Table 4.3 Sequence of instructions for examining power in the upper limb. Ax, axillary nerve; L, lateral; Md, median nerve; MI, medial; MS, musculoskeletal nerve; P, posterior; R, radial nerve; U, ulnar nerve

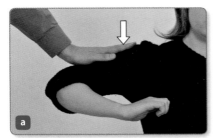

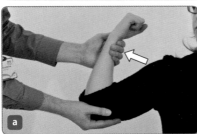

Figure 4.5 Assessment of the power of the axillary and musculoskeletal nerves. (a) Deltoid, C5/6, axillary. (b) Biceps, C5/6, musculoskeletal.

Note that there is some variation in nerve root and plexus contributions to peripheral nerves.

Testing muscle strength

To test muscle strength, firstly, instruct, demonstrate or move the patient's limb into the position where the muscle being tested is 'isolated' and needs to be active in order to maintain that position (e.g. the 'boxer' position to test biceps brachii). Next tell the patient 'Don't let me move your arm/hand/thumb, etc.' Attempt to overcome the muscle.

If the patient is too weak to maintain the muscle in the initial position, reposition the limb so that the muscle can contract without fighting against gravity, e.g. if the patient cannot contract biceps with the arm hanging by their side, hold the elbow and forearm up so that they can attempt to contract it in the horizontal plane. If too weak still, observe for any flicker of a movement in the muscle.

Grade the muscle strength.

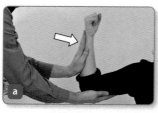

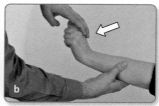

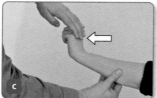

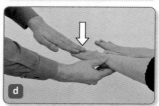

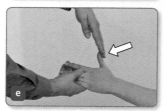

Figure 4.6 Assessment of the power of the radial nerve. (a) Triceps, C7, radial. (b) Extensor carpi radialis longus, C6, radial. (c) Extensor carpi ulnaris, C7, radial. (d) Extensor digitorum, C7, radial. (e) Extensor pollicis brevis, C7, radial.

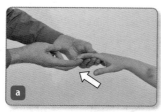

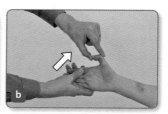

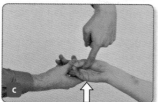

Figure 4.7 Assessment of the power of the median nerve. (a) Flexor digitorum profundus I and II, C8, median. (b) Flexor pollicis longus, C8, median. (c) Opponens pollicis, T1, median.

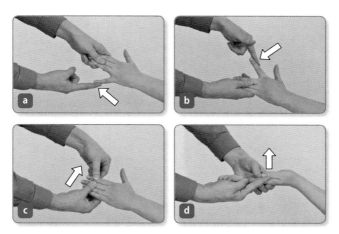

Figure 4.8 Assessment of the power of the ulnar nerve. (a) Flexor carpi ulnaris, C8, ulnar. (b) First dorsal interosseous, T1, ulnar. (c) Second palmar interosseous, T1, ulnar. (d) Adductor pollicis, T1, ulnar.

Key differential diagnoses
It is helpful to divide weakness into either flaccid (reduced tone) or spastic (increased tone) weakness.

Flaccid weakness
Flaccid weakness can be caused by:
- **myopathy**: proximal weakness is classic for most muscle diseases. An exception is inclusion body myositis, which occurs in the over 50s and presents with progressive distal arm and proximal leg weakness
- **neuromuscular junction**: diseases affecting the neuro-muscular junction include myasthenia gravis and Lambert–Eaton myasthenic syndrome (**Table 4.4**)
- **neuropathy**: flaccid weakness distal to the portion of the nerve affected. The longer a nerve is the more likely it is to be affected by a systemic process (e.g. inflammation, vasculitis, diabetes). This means that neuropathies are usually length dependent, and that the more distal muscles are affected

Clinical features	MG	LEMS
Weakness	Fluctuating, flaccid	Insidious, flaccid
Muscles affected	Ocular, bulbar, respiratory	Proximal limb muscles
Associated conditions	Thymoma Thymic hyperplasia	Small cell lung cancer (60%) Autoimmune disease
Antibodies	Anti-nicotinic acetylcholine receptors, anti-MuSK	Anti-P/Q type voltage-gated calcium channels
Effect of repeated muscle contraction	Fatigability	May be improvement
Slow repetitive nerve stimulation	Progressive decrement in CMAP	Progressive decrement in CMAP
Fast repetitive nerve stimulation	Progressive decrement in CMAP	Increase in CMAP (facilitation)
Other features	–	Autonomic dysfunction
Main treatments	Cholinesterase inhibitors Thymectomy Immunosuppression	Tumour removal 3,4-diaminopyridine Immunosuppression

Table 4.4 Summary of key clinical and laboratory features of myasthenia gravis (MG) and Lambert–Eaton myasthenic syndrome (LEMS). CMAP, compound muscle action potential

first. Localised nerve entrapment gives rise to characteristic patterns of weakness
• **radiculopathy**: damage to the cervical spinal or motor nerve roots will cause radicular pain and weakness in the muscles innervated from that level. The typical features of cervical radiculopathies are shown in **Table 4.5**

Spastic weakness

The causes of spastic weakness are:
• **spinal cord injury**: flaccid weakness occurs at the level of the injury due to damage to the exiting motor neuron itself; however, this may be very difficult to detect clinically because

Intervertebral disc affected (between vertebrae)	Spinal root affected	Pain/ sensory changes	Motor deficit	Reflex lost
C4 (C4 and C5)	C5	Shoulder, lateral upper arm	Deltoid, supraspinatus, infraspinatus	Supinator
C5 (C5 and C6)	C6	Lateral aspect of the forearm, thumb, forefinger	Biceps, brachioradialis	Biceps
C6 (C6 and C7)	C7	Dorsal aspect of the forearm, middle finger	Triceps, extensor muscles of wrist and fingers	Triceps
C7 (C7 and T1)	C8	4th and 5th digits and medial aspect of the palm	Intrinsic muscles of the hand, thumb flexor	–

Table 4.5 Clinical features of cervical intervertebral disc herniations

the damaged area may be quite small. Muscles innervated from the spinal cord below the level will have increased tone but be weak or completely paralysed. This is more obvious clinically because all of the cord below the lesion is affected

- **cortical lesions**: increased tone in the contralateral muscles. Typically, the arm extensors become weaker than the arm flexors, leading to an adducted arm, flexed at the elbow and the wrist

What happens next?

If there is any suggestion of a nerve or root lesion, examine the brachial plexus to further localise the lesion. **Table 4.6** shows the relevant muscles, nerves, plexus and roots to test.

Then, move on to test the reflexes.

Instruction	Muscle	Nerve	Plexus	Main root
Put your hand behind your back and push out	Rhomboids	Dorsal scapular	Superior trunk	C5
Lift your arm up to the side and push forward	Pectoralis major, clavicular head	Lateral pectoral	Lateral cord	C5
Lift your arm up to the side and push down	Subscapular	Teres major	Posterior cord	C5/6/7
Pull your elbows into your waist and turn your arms out	Infraspinatus	Suprascapular	Superior trunk	C5
Pull your elbows into your waist	Pectoralis major, sternocostal head	Lateral and medial pectoral	Lateral cord and inferior trunk	C6/7
Push your hands out in front	Serratus anterior	Long thoracic	Superior and middle trunks	C5/6/7
Cough for me	Latissimus dorsi	Thoracodorsal	Posterior cord	C7

Table 4.6 Instructions for examining power in the brachial plexus

4.7 Reflexes

Objective

This part of the examination is used to elicit reflexes and determine whether they are absent, reduced, normal or increased (hyper-reflexic).

Approach

Various muscle tendons are tapped to test their reflexes (**Figure 4.9**). The patient is positioned with their hands on their lap so that the upper limb muscles are relaxed and elbows slightly bent.

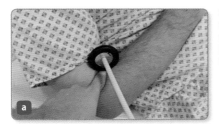

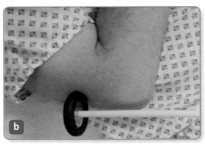

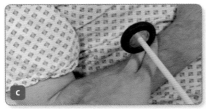

Figure 4.9 Reflexes of the upper limb. Sites to tap tendon hammer: (a) biceps, (b) triceps, (c) supinator.

Equipment
Reflex testing requires a tendon hammer.

Sequence
Tricep, bicep and supinator reflexes should be tested:

1. tap the tendon of biceps on each arm (C6) (**Figure 4.9a**)
2. tap the tendon of triceps on each arm (C7) (**Figure 4.9b**)
3. tap the tendon of supinator on each arm (C5) (**Figure 4.9c**)
4. if any reflex cannot be elicited, ask the patient to clench their teeth tight and then retest the reflex (reinforcement)

Key differential diagnoses

1. an absent or reduced reflex is one where a reflex is not elicited after reinforcement. This suggests a LMN lesion, but it
   may be normal in athletic individuals
2. hyper-reflexia suggests an UMN lesion. It may be present in
   anxious individuals

What happens next?

The next step is to test co-ordination.

4.8 Co-ordination

Sequence

To assess co-ordination in the upper limb:

1. ask the patient to 'Touch your nose with your right index
   finger'
2. ask them to 'Touch my finger with yours' while holding your
   finger at a distance forcing them to fully extend their arm
3. then ask them to 'Go back and forth quickly'
4. observe for any past pointing or intention tremor
5. repeat on other arm
6. ask the patient to 'Clap your right hand on top of your left'
7. when they start clapping, say 'Now flip your hand over each
   time you clap'
8. observe how quickly and smoothly they manage this

To properly assess for dysmetria or an intention tremor, ensure
the patient fully extends their arm when performing the nose-
finger test.

Key differential diagnoses

Poor co-ordination usually reflects cerebellar injury or, less commonly, a marked loss of proprioception. The following features
suggest a cerebellar lesion:

- **dysmetria**: overshooting target
- **intention tremor**: tremor beginning as finger approaches
  target
- **dysdiodochokinesia**: disorganised clapping movements

What happens next?
Finally, move on to test sensation.

4.9 Sensation

Objective
The purpose of this part of the examination is to assess the sensory function of the peripheral nerves, nerve roots and spinal cord supplying the upper limbs.

Approach
The patient has their sensation tested with their outer garments removed. Inform the patient that you are going to test their sense of touch in a number of ways, including with a dull pin tip that will not break their skin. Tell them that you are going to ask them whether the PP is sharp or dull and to compare it between sides.
   The principles of the sensory examination are to:
- start distally and work proximally
- test each major peripheral nerve
- test each major dermatome
- test both lateral and dorsal columns of the spinal cord
- map out any area of sensory change encountered

Equipment
This requires an examination pin, tuning fork and universal containers with hot and cold water.

Sequence
Test the function of the lateral and dorsal columns in turn.

Lateral columns
These are tested with either PP (pain) or hot and cold water (T°C):
1. touch the patient's sternum or forehead with the tip of the examination pin to show the patient what it feels like
2. touch each of the areas shown in **Figure 4.10**

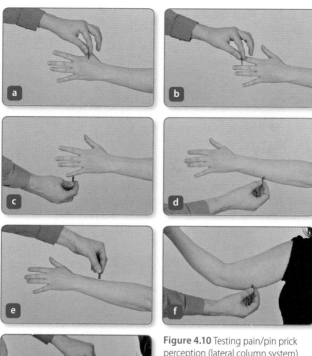

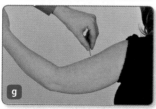

Figure 4.10 Testing pain/pin prick perception (lateral column system). An examination pin is touched gently against the skin at key locations: (a) radial nerve, C6; (b) median nerve, C7; (c) ulnar nerve, C8; (d) T1; (e) C6; (f) T2; (g) C5. The patient is asked whether it feels sharp. Temperature perception can be tested at the same sites with hot or cold water-filled universal containers.

3. repeat on the other side
4. if there are any abnormalities, repeat on the other side asking the patient to tell you if it feels the same on both sides
5. if there are any abnormalities, move in a proximal direction and retest until sensation returns to normal

6. in place of PP you can use hot and cold water in universal containers, touching the skin in the above sequence, asking if it is hot or cold

Dorsal columns

These are tested with a tuning fork (vibration) or joint movement (JPS).

Vibration

To examine vibration sense:

1. tap the tuning fork
2. place on the patient's clavicle and tell the patient 'This is what it feels like, can you feel it buzzing?'
3. tap before each placement
4. place the tuning fork on a bony prominence in each of the major dermatomes as shown in **Figure 4.11**
5. repeat on other side
6. if there are any abnormalities, repeat on the other side asking the patient to tell you if it feels the same on both sides
7. if there are any abnormalities, move in a proximal direction and retest until sensation returns to normal

Proprioception

Alternatively, in place of vibration you can test proprioception by moving joints (**Figure 4.12**):

1. isolate the joint by placing fingers proximally and distally
2. ask the patient to close their eyes and tell you if the joint moves up or down

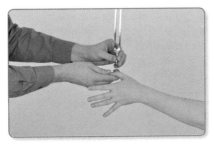

Figure 4.11 Testing vibration sense (dorsal column system). A vibrating tuning fork is placed onto a joint or bony prominent and the patient asked whether they perceive the vibration.

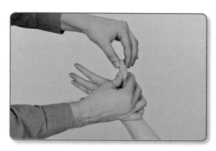

Figure 4.12 Technique for testing for joint position sense in the upper limb.

3. move the joint up or down – normally even tiny movements are appreciated
4. take care to place fingers to the sides of the joints rather than on top as you will otherwise stimulate pressure receptors rather than joint position sense
5. start at the distal joints and move proximally until there is normal perception of movement

Key differential diagnoses

These include:

- **mononeuropathy**: loss of multiple modalities in the distribution of a recognisable peripheral nerve
- **polyneuropathy**: typically, this is length dependent (distal nerves are affected first), leading to a 'glove-and-stocking' loss of sensation. It often affects multiple modalities
- **brachial plexopathy**: usually multiple modalities. The distribution may look like multiple peripheral nerves or nerve roots
- **radiculopathy**: usually multiple modalities. The distribution is in the pattern of one or more recognisable dermatomes. Often, there is spontaneous pain in the affected dermatome or pain elicited by PP or a vibrating fork

Cord syndrome	Pain and temperature loss	JPS and vibration loss	Motor weakness
Complete	Bilateral below lesion	Bilateral below lesion	Severe Bilateral below lesion
Anterior	Bilateral below lesion	Intact	Severe Bilateral below lesion
Posterior	Intact	Bilateral below lesion	Milder Bilateral below lesion
Lateral	Contralateral below lesion	Ipsilateral below lesion	Mild or severe Ipsilateral below lesion
Central	Bilateral at level of lesion	Intact	Unaffected until advanced

Table 4.7 Summary of clinical features of spinal cord syndromes. JPS, joint position sense

- **myelopathy**: lesions in the spinal cord itself can give rise to more complex sensory findings (**Figure 4.4**). Features suggestive of a spinal lesion include: (1) dissociated sensory loss, i.e. differential loss of dorsal column and lateral column modalities, and (2) sensory level, i.e. a point above which sensation returns to normal

Table 4.7 summarises the various spinal cord syndromes.

What happens next?
Move on to examine the lower limbs.

4.10 System summary

A summary of upper limb examination is given in **Table 4.8**.

Inspection	Syndrome, posture, fasciculations, wasting, pronator drift
Tone	Spasticity, flaccid, cog-wheeling
Power	Deltoid Bicep Tricep Extensor carpi radialis longus Extensor carpi ulnaris Extensor digitorum Extensor pollicis longus Pronator teres Flexor digitorum profundus I and II Flexor pollicis longus Opponens pollicis Flexor carpi ulnaris 1st dorsal interosseous 2nd palmar interosseous Adductor pollicis
Reflexes	Tricep, bicep, brachioradialis
Co-ordination	Finger nose, dysdiodochokinesia
Sensation	Pin-prick and vibration
	Radial, medial, ulnar nerves
	Dermatomes

Table 4.8 Examination of the upper limb

Lower limb

5.1 Objectives

Examination of the lower limb is very similar in approach to that of the upper limb. The same sequence of examining tone, power, reflexes, co-ordination and sensation is followed and the same general rules about upper motor neuron (UMN) and lower motor neuron (LMN) lesions and patterns of spinal cord injury apply.

5.2 Anatomy and physiology review

Table 5.1 summarises the motor functions of the major nerves in the lower limb. Think of them as four major nerves: gluteal, femoral, obturator and sciatic. The sciatic can be further subdivided into three: the proximal portion supplying the hamstrings; the common peroneal nerve supplying the foot extensors; and the tibial nerve supplying the foot flexors.

The pudendal nerve is relatively small but is important in the control of bowel and bladder function. It originates from neurons in Onuf's nucleus in the spinal cord and is derived from the roots of S2–4. It carries sensory information from the perineum and perianal region and controls the anal and bladder sphincters.

Clinical insight

Testing the function of the pudendal nerve is important when assessing for possible cauda equina syndrome. This is compression of the cauda equina, usually from a prolapsed disc below L4. Compression of S2–4 will disrupt the function of the pudendal nerve, leading to:

- loss of anal tone: assessed per rectum
- bladder dysfunction: usually retention with overflow incontinence; assessed by postvoiding bladder scan and catheterisation
- saddle anaesthesia: assessed by blunt pin-prick
- sexual dysfunction (e.g. erectile dysfunction; assessed in the history)

Nerve	Root	Key muscles	Muscle action
Gluteal	L4/5	Gluteus maximus Gluteus medius and minimus	Hip extension Internal rotation of thigh and hip abduction
Femoral	L1/2 L3/4	Iliacus Quadriceps femoris	Hip flexion Knee extension
Obturator	L2/3	Adductor brevis, longus and magnus, gracilis	Adduction of lower limb
Sciatic: proximal portion	S1	'Hamstrings'	Knee flexion
Sciatic: common peroneal	L5/S1 L4 L5/S1	Peroneus longus and brevis Tibialis anterior Extensor digitorum longus and brevis Extensor hallucis longus	Eversion of the foot Dorsiflexion of the foot Dorsiflexion of the toes Dorsiflexion of the distal phalanx of the big toe
Sciatic: tibial nerve	S1/2 L4/5 S1/2 S1/2	Gastrocnemius Tibialis posterior Flexor digitorum and hallucis longus Small muscles of the foot	Plantarflexion of the foot Inversion of the foot Flexion of the toes 'Cupping' of the toes

Table 5.1 Summary of the major motor functions of the peripheral nerves in the lower limb

Upper and lower motor neurons
Lesions affecting the lower limb can be divided into UMN and LMN lesions, as shown in **Figure 4.2**.

Gluteal nerve
Key anatomy of the gluteal nerve:
- The superior gluteal nerve supplies gluteus medius (GluMe) and minimus (GluMi); the inferior gluteal nerve supplies gluteus maximus (GluMax)
- roots L4/5
- sensory: none
- motor: GluMax is a powerful hip extensor; GluMe and GluMi internally rotate and abduct the thigh

Femoral nerve

Key anatomy of the femoral nerve:

- roots: L1–4
- sensory: the medial and intermediate cutaneous nerves of the thigh supply sensation to the anterior aspect of the thigh and knee and the medial aspect of the knee; the saphenous nerve supplies sensation to the medial aspect of the lower leg to the ankle
- motor: iliacus is a powerful hip flexor; the quadriceps extend the knee

> ### Clinical insight
>
> Femoral neuropathy:
>
> - weakness of hip flexion and knee extension
> - knee often 'gives way' when standing or walking
> - loss of reflex at the knee
> - sensory loss over the anterior thigh and knee and medial aspect of the lower leg
> - causes: diabetes, hip or pelvis fractures, femoral artery catheterisation, and compression from retroperitoneal tumours

Obturator nerve

Key anatomy of the obturator nerve:

- roots: L2/3
- sensory: supplies sensation to the medial aspect of the thigh
- motor: adductors of the lower limb

Sciatic nerve

Key anatomical features of the proximal portion (from the origin to the division of the tibial and common peroneal nerves):

- roots: L5/S1/S2
- sensory: the posterior cutaneous nerve of the thigh originates at the same level as, and travels close by, the sciatic nerve. It supplies the posterior aspect of the thigh
- motor: the 'hamstrings' flex the knee

Common peroneal nerve

The common peroneal nerve gives rise to the superficial and deep peroneal nerves at the head of the fibula. Key anatomical features include:

- roots: L4/L5/S1

- sensory: superficial peroneal supplies the dorsum of the foot except the web space between the first and second toes, which is supplied by the deep peroneal nerve
- motor: the superficial peroneal supplies peroneus longus and brevis (foot eversion); the deep peroneal supplies tibialis anterior (foot dorsiflexion), extensor digitorum longus and brevis (toe dorsiflexion), and extensor hallucis longus (dorsiflexes the distal phalanx of the great toe)

Tibial nerve

Key anatomical features of the tibial nerve:

- roots: L4–S2
- sensory: the sural nerve and the plantar nerves supply the lateral aspect and the sole of the foot, respectively
- motor: gastrocnemius plantarflexes the foot; tibialis posterior inverts the foot; flexor digitorum and hallucis longus flex the toes; the small muscles of the foot 'cup' the toes

Clinical insight

Common peroneal neuropathy:

- foot drop, weak foot eversion but spared inversion
- sensory loss over the dorsum of the foot and anterior and lateral aspects of the leg
- causes: trauma at the head of the fibula, chronic crossing of legs, prolonged squatting, knee trauma

Clinical insight

Tibial neuropathy:

- weakness of plantarflexion
- loss of sensation on the sole of the foot
- causes: trauma or surgery in the popliteal fossa or ankle, entrapment at the posterior tarsal tunnel (pain and numbness at the ankle and sole), diabetes

The lumbosacral plexus

The lumbosacral plexus is the lower limb equivalent of the brachial plexus. The anatomy is more complex than in the brachial plexus and a working knowledge of it is a specialist area. Retroperitoneal tumours can cause compressive lesions, as can local nerve infarction or inflammation.

Intervertebral discs

Key anatomy of intervertebral discs:
- vertebral bodies are named in sequence: C1–C8, T1–T12, L1–L5 and S1–S5
- intervertebral discs are named after the vertebral body above and below: e.g. the L4/5 disc occurs between L4 and L5
- in the cervical region, spinal roots C1–7 exit above their named vertebral body (i.e. the C4 root exits above the C4 body, at the C3/4 disc) and root C8 exits below C7 (there is no C8 vertebral body)
- in the thoracic and lumbar regions the roots exit below their named vertebral body (i.e. the L5 root exits below L5, at the L5/S1 disc)

> ## Clinical insight
>
> Sciatic neuropathy:
> - weakness of knee flexion
> - weakness of dorsiflexion and plantarflexion of ankle
> - foot drop, weakness of foot inversion and eversion
> - loss of ankle reflex
> - loss of sensation over the sole and dorsum of the foot, with sparing of the medial aspect
> - causes: hip surgery or fracture, compression from tumour or haemorrhage, entrapment at the piriformis muscle, diabetes, inflammation, and infection

5.3 Clinical features and pathophysiology

The important general abnormal findings for general inspection, patterns of weakness and sensory disturbance for the lower limb are the same as described for the upper limb in Chapter 4 (see page 92).

Intervertebral disc prolapse

The relation between the prolapsed disc level, exiting nerve root at that level, and the root compressed when the disc prolapses is shown in **Table 5.2**.

Cervical and thoracic disc prolapse

Discs prolapse posterolaterally and compress the nerve root exiting at that same level, i.e. a C5/6 disc prolapse compresses the exiting C6 root. Thoracic disc prolapses are rare.

Prolapsed disc	Exiting root	Compressed root
C1/2	C2	C2
C2/3	C3	C3
C3/4	C4	C4
C4/5	C5	C5
C5/6	C6	C6
C6/7	C7	C7
C7/T1	C8	C8
L1/2	L1	L2
L2/3	L2	L3
L3/4	L3	L4
L4/5	L4	L5
L5/S1	L5	S1

Table 5.2 Relation between the level of the prolapsed disc, the nerve root which exits at that level, and the root compressed by the prolapse

Lumbar disc prolapse

These also usually prolapse posterolaterally. Owing to the relative height of the lumbar vertebral bodies, a prolapsed lumbar disc does not compress the nerve root exiting at the same level (e.g. an L5/S1 disc prolapse does not compress the exiting L5 disc) because the nerve root exits higher than the prolapse. Instead, it compresses the descending nerve root that exits at the next level (e.g. an L5/S1 disc prolapse compresses the descending S1 root, which exits at S1/2).

Clinical insight

Disc prolapses: an easy way to remember the disc levels, exiting roots and which root is compressed is:

- the compressed root is always the second number in the disc level name (e.g. L2/3 disc herniation compresses root L3; C4/5 disc herniation compresses root C5)
- the exiting root is the second number for cervical discs (at the C4/5 disc level the C5 root exits) but the first number for lumbar discs (at the L2/3 disc level the L2 root exits)

5.4 General observations

Objective
The purpose of this part of the examination is to identify any characteristic features of neurological disease affecting the lower limbs.

Approach
Ask the patient to remove their outer garments.

Sequence
In generally assessing the lower limb, observe from in front and then behind. Look for:
1. **asymmetry** in posture of the lower limb
2. **muscle wasting,** particularly tibialis anterior and the quadriceps
3. **foot deformities** such as pes cavus
4. **fasciculations**: these may be evident only after prolonged observation

Key findings
These include:
- abnormal posture of one leg: dystonia, simple partial seizure, hemiplegia
- muscle wasting: LMN lesions lead to denervation of muscle and muscle atrophy. Long-standing UMN lesions can eventually cause wasting through disuse
- foot deformities: may point to a hereditary sensorimotor neuropathy
- fasciculations: these may be benign (e.g. young patient, after exercise) or from motor neuron disease or any cause of denervation (i.e. LMN lesion)

What happens next?
The next step is to examine tone.

5.5 Tone

Objective
The aim of this part of the examination is to identify any pathologically increased or decreased tone.

Sequence
To examine tone:
1. ask the patient to lie flat on the couch
2. roll their legs at the thigh, watching the ankle
3. pull up sharply behind the knee, dragging the heel up the couch
4. normally, the foot will wiggle quite freely at the ankle when you roll the thighs and the ankle will drag up the surface of the couch when the knee is jerked up.

Key findings
Tone can be found to be increased or decreased:
- **increased tone** is suggested by an ankle that appears fixed in position when the thigh is rolled or when the heel comes off the couch upon jerking the knee. This indicates increased tonic activation of an intact LMN, i.e. an UMN lesion. It can be pathological, normal or from anxiety
- **reduced tone** indicates decreased tonic activation of muscles. Hyperacute UMN lesions can sometimes cause flaccid weakness (e.g. acute stroke). Generally, this indicates a LMN lesion

What happens next?
Next, examine power.

5.6 Power

Objective
This part of the assessment examines the strength of individual muscles, thereby assessing muscle function and indirectly peripheral nerve, nerve root, spinal cord and cortical function.

Approach

The general principles of assessing power in the upper limb (Chapter 4, see page 95) apply here too. The aim is to grade the muscle strength (see **Table 4.2**).

Sequence

The sequence tests the muscles in turn in a logical order to assess a number of muscles from each major peripheral nerve and nerve root. The verbal instructions are given in **Table 5.3**, as is the muscle being tested, the innervating nerve and the major root. **Figures 5.1–5.4** demonstrate the key muscles to test. There is some variation in nerve root contributions to peripheral nerves.

Key findings
UMN lesion

The following findings may help differentiate between lesions in the cortex or spinal cord:

- a **hemispheric cortical lesion** tends to result in a weak, spastic lower limb with the leg held in extension at the hip, knee and ankle
- a **spinal lesion** will cause UMN signs below the level affected. The examiner will be able to 'get above the lesion', e.g. a lesion at T2 will cause UMN signs in the legs but a normal examination of the arms
- a spinal lesion also theoretically causes LMN signs at the level of the lesion since it will destroy the cell body of the motor neurons at this level. However, this may be difficult to detect clinically

LMN lesion

The differential diagnosis is fairly wide and is between The following may help differentiate between muscle, mononeuropathy, polyneuropathy, plexus and root lesions.:

- **myopathy**. This will give the following:
  - LMN signs
  - proximal weakness with difficulty standing or squatting

Instruction	Muscle	Muscle action	Nerve	Root
Lift your leg up	Iliacus/psoas major	Hip flexion	Femoral	L1/2
Push your leg into the couch	Gluteus maximus	Extension at the hip	Inferior gluteal	L5/S1
Don't let me separate your legs	Adductors	Adduction at the hip	Obturator	L2/3
Bend your knee, don't let me turn your leg out	Gluteus medius and minimus	Internal rotation of the thigh	Superior gluteal	L4/5
Bend your knee, don't let me bend it more	Quadriceps	Extension at the knee	Femoral	L3/4
Bend your knee, don't let me straighten it	Hamstrings	Flexion at the knee	Sciatic	S1
Push your foot down	Gastrocnemius	Plantarflexion at the ankle	Tibial	S1/2
Turn your foot in	Tibialis posterior	Inversion of the foot	Tibial	L4/5
Curl your toes	Small muscles of the foot	Cupping of the foot	Tibial	S1/2
Point your foot towards your head	Tibialis anterior	Dorsiflexion at the ankle	Deep peroneal	L4
Point your big toe towards your head	Extensor hallucis longus	Extension of the toe	Deep peroneal	L5
Turn your foot out	Peroneus longus and brevis	Eversion of the foot	Superficial peroneal	L5/S1

Table 5.3 For each instruction ask the patient to position their limb as described and tell them 'Don't let me move it' before applying an antagonistic force

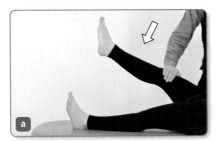

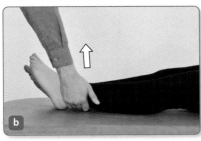

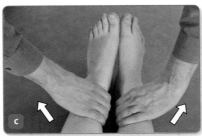

Figure 5.1 Assessment of power around the hip. The arrow indicates the direction of force exerted by the examiner. (a) Iliacus, L1/2, femoral. (b) Gluteus maximus, L5/S1, inferior gluteal. (c) Adductors, L2/3, obturator.

- usually symmetrical
- often also tender muscles
- **mononeuropathies** show weakness in a pattern attributable to a single nerve
- **polyneuropathies** show weakness in muscles innervated by several peripheral nerves. Typically, distal is worse than proximal and it is usually symmetrical
- **sacral plexopathies** are essentially unilateral polyneuropathies with muscles affected from multiple nerves

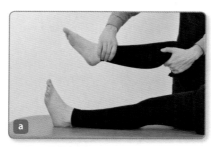

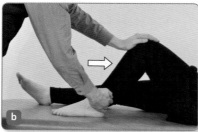

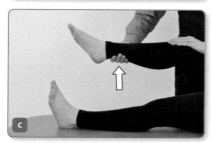

Figure 5.2 Assessment of power around the knee. The arrow indicates the direction of force exerted by the examiner. (a) Gluteus medius and minimus, L4/5, superior gluteal. (b) Quadriceps, L3/4, femoral. (c) Hamstring, S1, sciatic.

- a **root lesion** is most readily identified by the distribution of pain; however, if there is involvement of the ventral or spinal root, weakness will also be seen. This will be in muscles not restricted to a single peripheral nerve but to a recognisable spinal level

What happens next?

Move on to test the reflexes.

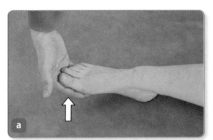

Figure 5.3 Assessment of power of the muscles of the tibial nerve. The arrow indicates the direction of force exerted by the examiner. (a) Gastrocnemius, S1/2, tibial. (b) Tibialis posterior, L4/5, tibial. (c) Small muscles of the foot, S1/2, tibial.

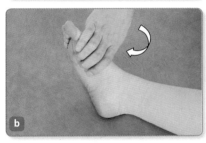

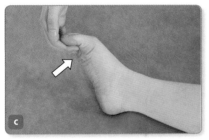

5.7 Reflexes

Objective

The aim of this part of the examination is to elicit reflexes and determine whether they are absent, reduced, normal or increased (hyper-reflexic).

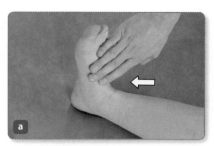

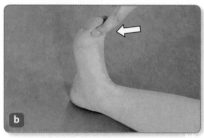

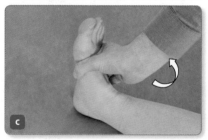

Figure 5.4 Assessment of power of the muscles of the peroneal nerve. The arrow indicates the direction of force exerted by the examiner. (a) Tibialis anterior, L4, deep peroneal. (b) Extensor hallucis longus, L5, deep peroneal. (c) Peroneus longus and brevis, L5/S1, superficial peroneal.

Approach

During the examination, various muscle tendons are tapped to test their reflexes.

Equipment

A tendon hammer is required.

Sequence

To assess lower limb reflexes and clonus:

1. ask the patient to lie flat on the couch
2. take the weight of each leg in turn by lifting under the knee
3. tap the patellar tendon for the knee jerk (L3/4) (**Figure 5.5a**)
4. with legs flat tap the medial aspect of the knee where the adductors attach; watch both legs for adduction: crossed adductor reflex (L2–5)
5. flex the knee slightly, turn the foot outward and hold it dorsiflexed, tap the Achilles tendon: the ankle jerk (**Figure 5.5b** and **c**) (S1/2)
6. stroke the lateral sole of the foot upwards and across to the ball of the foot, observing the initial direction of movement of the great toe: the plantar reflex (**Figure 5.6**)
7. check for clonus by:
   - gently rolling the ankle briefly then forcefully holding it dorsiflexed
   - observe any rhythmic plantarflexion of the ankle
   - more than four beats is likely to be pathological

Clinical insight

The hallmark of nerve root disease is the progression from radicular pain, through radicular sensory loss to radicular weakness. Radicular pain is usually the first symptom of nerve root compression. The radiation of the pain usually indicates the level of origin:

Nerve root affected	Pain radiation
C5	Shoulder
C6	Lateral forearm and thumb
C7	Dorsum of hand and middle finger
C8	Medial forearm, medial two fingers
L1	Groin
L2	Medial thigh
L3	Knee
L4	Inner calf
L5	Outer calf and great toe
S1	Lateral foot and sole
S2	Posterior thigh

Clinical insight

Getting above the lesion: when signs of weakness (or sensory disturbance) are found in the arms or legs a helpful strategy is to attempt to 'get above the lesion'. This means finding the level of the nervous system above which function is normal. Since lesions in the central nervous system or peripheral nervous system will cause weakness or sensory disturbance **distally,** the level at which power returns to normal indicates that the lesion is below this.

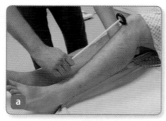

Figure 5.5 Reflexes of the lower limb. How to test the (a) knee jerk, and (b) and (c) ankle jerk.

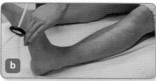

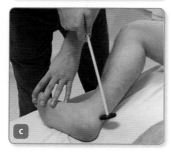

8. if any reflex cannot be elicited, ask the patient to grip their hands together and pull hard (reinforcement) as you test

Key findings

These are:

*   **absent or reduced** knee or ankle reflex: this is only considered absent if the reflex is not elicited after reinforcement. It indicates a LMN lesion, but may be normal in athletic individuals
*   **hyper-reflexia**: indicates an UMN lesion, but may be present in anxious individuals
*   **crossed adductor** reflex present; this is abnormal and indicates an UMN lesion

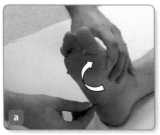
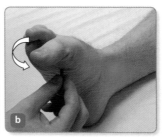
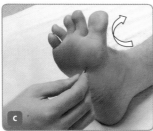

Figure 5.6 Testing the plantar reflex. (a) Stroking the sole of the foot (white arrow) elicits either (b) normal plantar flexion of the great toe or (c) abnormal dorsiflexion of the great toe and fanning of the toes.

- **flexor plantar** reflex (downward): this is normal
- **extensor plantar** reflex (upward): indicates an UMN lesion
- **persistent clonus**: indicates an UMN lesion

What happens next?

The next stage is to test co-ordination.

5.8 Co-ordination

Objective

The next step is to assess the co-ordination of the lower limb.

Sequence

Ask the patient to:
1. 'lift your heel off the couch'
2. 'touch it to your other knee'
3. 'run it down your shin'
4. 'lift it up and do it again'
5. 'tap out a rhythm with your heel'

Key findings

Poor co-ordination usually reflects cerebellar injury or a marked loss of proprioception. The following features suggest a cerebellar lesion:

- **dysmetria**: overshooting the target
- **intention tremor**: tremor beginning as the heel approaches the target
- **dysdiodochokinesia**: disorganised movements

Proprioceptive loss can also cause tremor or dysmetria but this tends to be less dramatic.

What happens next?

The final step in this part of the examination is to test sensation.

5.9 Sensation

Objective

The purpose of the final step in this part of the examination is to assess the sensory function of the peripheral nerves, nerve roots and spinal cord supplying the lower limb.

Approach

Sensation is tested with the patient's outer garments removed. Inform the patient that you are going to test the sense of touch in a number of ways, including with a dull pin tip that will not break their skin. Tell them that you are going to ask them whether the pin-prick is sharp or dull and to compare it between sides.

The principles of the sensory examination are to:

- start distally and work proximally
- test each major peripheral nerve
- test each major dermatome (see **Figure 4.1** for dermatomes of the lower limb)
- test both lateral and dorsal columns of the spinal cord
- map out any area of sensory change encountered

Equipment

This requires an examination pin, tuning fork and universal containers with hot and cold water.

Sequence

Test the function of the lateral and dorsal columns in turn.

Lateral columns

These are tested with either pin-prick (PP) (pain) or hot and cold water [temperature (T)]:

1. touch the patient's sternum or forehead with the tip of the examination pin to show the patient what it feels like
2. touch each of the areas in **Figure 5.7** and ask 'Does it feel sharp or dull?'
3. this is usually sufficient to screen in a general examination. However, if cauda equina syndrome is suspected, also ensure to check perianal and perineal sensation:
   - buttocks (inferior lateral clunical nerve; S3)
   - perianal (pudendal nerve; S4/5)
4. if there is an area of abnormal sensation that persists up to L4, higher dermatomes must be tested until an area of normal sensation has been detected, i.e. the upper limit of the lesion has been detected. For this, test:
   - knee (L3)
   - thigh (L2)
   - hips (L1)
   - level of the umbilicus (T10)
   - halfway between the umbilicus and nipples (T7)
   - level of the nipples (T4)
   - lower border of the clavicle (T2)
5. repeat on the other side
6. if there is an abnormality at a level, repeat on the other side asking the patient to say if it feels the same on both sides
7. in place of PP, you can use hot and cold water in universal containers, touching the skin in the above sequence, asking if it is hot or cold

Dorsal columns

These are tested with a tuning fork (vibration) or joint movement (JPS).

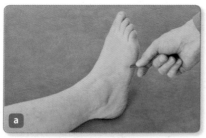

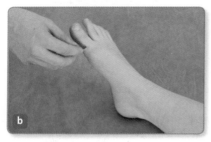

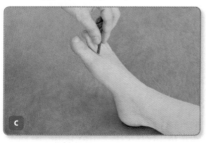

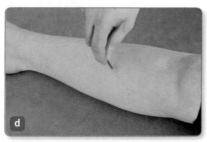

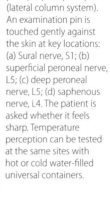

Figure 5.7 Testing pain/pin prick perception (lateral column system). An examination pin is touched gently against the skin at key locations: (a) Sural nerve, S1; (b) superficial peroneal nerve, L5; (c) deep peroneal nerve, L5; (d) saphenous nerve, L4. The patient is asked whether it feels sharp. Temperature perception can be tested at the same sites with hot or cold water-filled universal containers.

Vibration

To examine vibration sense:

1. tap the tuning fork
2. place on the patient's clavicle, or forehead if a high thoracic lesion is possible, and tell the patient 'This is what it feels like, can you feel it buzzing?'
3. tap before each placement
4. place the tuning fork on bony prominences in the key dermatomes, as shown in **Figure 5.8**
5. if there is an area of abnormal sensation that persists up to L1, higher dermatomes must be tested until an area of normal sensation has been detected, i.e. the upper limit of the lesion has been detected. For this, test:
   - rib at the level of the umbilicus (T10)
   - rib halfway between the umbilicus and nipples (T7)
   - rib at the level of the nipples (T4)
   - clavicle (T2)

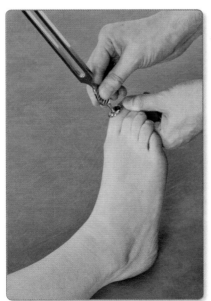

Figure 5.8 Testing vibration sense (dorsal column system). A vibrating tuning fork is placed onto a joint or bony prominent and the patient asked whether they perceive the vibration. (a) Sural nerve, S1; (b) superficial peroneal nerve, L5; (c) saphenous nerve, L4; (d) femoral nerve, L3; (e) hip, L1.

6. repeat on the other side
7. if there are any abnormalities, repeat on the other side asking the patient to tell you if it feels the same on both sides
8. if there are any abnormalities, move in a proximal direction and retest until sensation returns to normal

Proprioception

Alternatively, in place of vibration you can test proprioception by moving joints (**Figure 5.9**):

1. isolate the joint by placing fingers proximally and distally
2. ask the patient to close their eyes and tell you if the joint moves up or down
3. move the joint up or down: normally even tiny movements are appreciated
4. take care to place fingers to the sides of the joints rather than on top as you will otherwise stimulate pressure receptors rather than joint position sense
5. start at the distal joints and move proximally until the patient has normal perception of movement

Key findings

These include:

- **mononeuropathy**: loss of multiple modalities in the distribution of a recognisable peripheral nerve

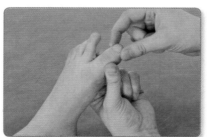

Figure 5.9 Position for testing for joint position sense in the lower limb.

- **polyneuropathy**: this will typically be length dependent, meaning that the distal nerves are affected first, which leads to a 'glove-and-stocking' loss of sensation. This often affects multiple modalities
- **sacral plexopathy**: usually multiple modalities. The distribution may look like multiple peripheral nerves or nerve roots
- **radiculopathy**: usually multiple modalities. The distribution is in the pattern of one or more recognisable dermatomes. Often, there is spontaneous pain in the affected dermatome or pain elicited by PP or vibrating fork
- **myelopathy**: lesions in the spinal cord itself can give rise to more complex sensory findings (see **Figure 4.4**). The following indicate a spinal cord lesion: (1) dissociated sensory loss, i.e. loss of only one dorsal column or lateral column modality, and (2) sensory level, i.e. a clear point on the patient's body below which sensation is lost and above which sensation returns to normal

See **Table 4.7** for a summary of the clinical features of cord syndromes.

What happens next?

Selecting the appropriate investigations depends primarily on the suspected location of the lesion:

- Lesions localising to the muscles or peripheral nerves should be investigated with nerve conduction studies
- Suspected nerve root or spinal cord lesions are best investigated with MRI of the spine to show soft-tissue injury, such as prolapsed discs and myelopathy
- A CT of the spine is helpful if significant bony disease (e.g. fracture) is suspected

5.10 System summary

Neurological examination of the lower limb is summarised in **Table 5.4**.

Inspection	Syndromes, posture, fasciculations, wasting, feet
Tone	Spastic, flaccid
Power	Gluteus maximus, adductors, iliacus, quadriceps, gluteus medius/gluteus minimis, hamstrings, gastrocnemius, tibialis posterior, small muscles of the foot, tibialis anterior, extensor hallucis longus, peroneus longus and brevis
Reflexes	Knee, crossed adductor, ankle, plantars, clonus
Co-ordination	Heel–shin, tap rhythm
Sensation	Pin-prick: (1) outer foot, great toe, medial tibia, knee, lateral thigh, popliteal fossa, buttocks, perianal, perineum; (2) thoracic region if indicated
	Vibration: (1) lateral malleolus, great toe, mid-tibia, tibial plateau, hip; (2) ribs and sternum if indicated

Table 5.4 Examination of the lower limb

Cerebellum

6.1 Objectives

The gross motor functions of the cerebellum are tested during several other stages of the neurological examination, e.g. in looking for nystagmus in the cranial nerve examination or testing co-ordination in the limb examination. Nonetheless, a systematic approach to examining cerebellar function is needed when the history or initial examination indicates cerebellar disease.

6.2 Anatomy and physiology review

The functions of the cerebellum remain incompletely understood. Its role in the fine control of movements is the most clinically relevant; however, it is also involved in a wide range of higher functions, including emotion and cognition.

The main clinical manifestations of cerebellar disease can be remembered by the acronym VANISHD: **V**ertigo, **A**taxia, **N**ystagmus, **I**ntention tremor, **S**peech disturbance, **H**ypotonia and **D**ysdiodokokinesia. This can also be used as the basis for an examination routine.

The cerebellum is located in the posterior fossa and contains over half of the neurons of the brain. It has a unique and uniform arrangement of cells that constitute basic circuits repeated many millions of times. It can be divided into different regions based on gross anatomy, which also corresponds to the origin of the major inputs and outputs.

The cerebellum forms the feed-forward control over movements, smoothing out movements initiated elsewhere and ensuring the intended movement is accurately performed. There are three anatomically distinct areas: the anterior lobe, the posterior lobe and the flocculonodular lobe (**Figure 6.1**). The cerebellum has three functionally distinct areas, each with distinct inputs and outputs:

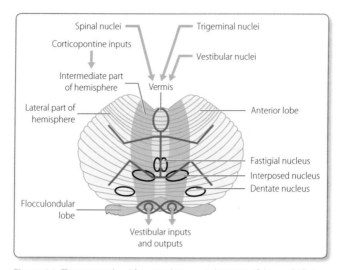

Figure 6.1 The structural and functional inputs and outputs of the cerebellum. Somatotopic organisation is shown in red: head, neck and axial movements are controlled by circuits in the midline of the cerebellum, and limb movements are controlled more laterally in the hemispheres and by vestibular and ocular circuits in the flocculonodular lobe.

- the **central vermis** receives spinal, trigeminal, vestibular and visual inputs and projects to regions controlling the axial trunk and head
- the **intermediate** part of the hemispheres receives mainly spinal and trigeminal inputs and projects to lateral descending systems of motor control of the trunk and limbs
- the **lateral** part of the hemispheres receives corticopontine inputs and projects to the motor and premotor cortices of the limbs and hands and feet

Each area is also associated with specific nuclei:
- the vermis with the fastigial nuclei
- the intermediate areas with the interposed nuclei
- the lateral areas with the dentate nuclei

The anatomical flocculonodular lobe receives mainly vestibular inputs and projects back to the vestibular nuclei and is closely involved in eye movements.

6.3 Clinical features and pathophysiology

Cerebellar disease from many causes tends to produce the same range of symptoms and signs. These can be remembered with the acronym VANISHD.

Vertigo

This is the illusory perception of movement – like 'stepping off a roundabout'. Patients may not be familiar with this meaning of the word, and so care should be taken to fully determine the nature of any dizziness, faintness or unsteadiness that they report.

Ataxia

Ataxia is objective dysfunction of balance or co-ordination. Ataxia is truncal when it affects the posture of the trunk. This is evident even while sitting upright. Appendicular ataxia is when a limb is affected. Ataxia may be evident on walking, when a patient will tend to fall to the affected side of a unilateral lesion.

Nystagmus

Nystagmus is the inability to maintain gaze fixation. There is a slow phase of eye movement away from the target followed by a rapid saccade to correct it. The direction

Guiding principles

Ataxia can be caused by any of:
- Cerebellar disease
- Peripheral nerve disease (proprioceptive fibre loss)
- Spinal cord disease (dorsal column loss)
- Vestibular disease

The associated symptoms and signs will help determine which it is.

Clinical insight

Peripheral nystagmus tends to be unilateral (i.e. it occurs mainly when looking in one direction) with the fast phase pointing away from the lesion. In central nystagmus, the fast phase tends to change so that it occurs in the direction of gaze.

of the fast phase is the direction of nystagmus (i.e. if the slow phase is to the left then the fast correction is back to the right and it is described as right-beating nystagmus).

Nystagmus may be normal (physiological) or abnormal from peripheral lesions (i.e. to the vestibular system) or central lesions. It can occur at rest; be gaze evoked; or be position evoked. Central lesions (e.g. in the cerebellum) tend to produce spontaneous nystagmus at rest, whereas peripheral lesions tend to be evoked by position. Nystagmus can be described as horizontal, vertical or rotational.

Intention tremor

This is a tremor that increases as the limb approaches the target. Similar symptoms such as dysmetria (overshooting or undershooting a target) and impaired check (failure to stop a limb movement appropriately) also commonly occur in cerebellar lesions.

Speech disturbance

Typically, cerebellar lesions result in a dysarthria with intact semantics. There may also be scanning speech in which there are pauses between words or syllables.

Hypotonia

Decreased tone can occur in acute cerebellar lesions.

Dysdiodochokinesia

This is the inability to accurately perform rapidly alternating movements. As with many of the clinical abnormalities of cerebellar disease, it is thought to be due to poor co-ordination of agonist and antagonist muscles.

6.4 General observations

Objective

The objective of general observation is to identify any gross signs of cerebellar disease and any potential causes.

Approach
The patient should undress to their undergarments.

Sequence
In generally assessing cerebellar function:
1. observe the patient from in front and then behind
2. look for foot deformities, hypothyroid facies or evidence of chronic liver disease
3. feel the pulse
4. auscultate the carotids
5. palpate the abdomen, particularly looking for an enlarged or irregular liver edge

Key findings
Key differentials include:
- pes cavus and cerebellar signs may indicate Friedreich's ataxia, an autosomal recessive genetic disorder
- atrial fibrillation or carotid bruits may indicate cerebrovascular disease as a cause of cerebellar disease
- hepatomegaly or evidence of chronic liver disease indicates chronic ethanol use as a cause of cerebellar disease
- craggy hepatomegaly indicates disseminated malignancy, which could include posterior fossa metastases or a paraneoplastic cerebellar syndrome.

What happens next?
Next, follow the VANISHD routine explained below.

6.5 VANISHD

Objective
The purpose is to systematically review the major clinical abnormalities found in cerebellar disease: **V**ertigo, **A**taxia, **N**ystagmus, **I**ntention tremor, **S**peech disturbance, **H**ypotonia and **D**ysdiodokokinesia.

Approach

Tell the patient that their ability to perform a range of movements will be assessed.

Sequence

Assess the patient for features of cerebellar dysfunction using the acronym VANISHD as a guide.

Vertigo

Vertigo is a symptom and therefore should have been clarified in the history.

Ataxia

To assess for ataxia:

1. ask the patient to sit upright in the chair with their back forward from the chair back
2. note any oscillations in the trunk, neck or head
3. ask them to stand. Note the position of their feet (i.e. any broad-based stance)
4. ask them to walk to the end of the room, turn and come back
5. note the pattern of the gait and whether they fall to one side

Nystagmus

Closely check for nystagmus:

1. ask them to sit again
2. ask them to look at your nose. Note any nystagmus in primary gaze
3. test their range of eye movements again, noting the presence and fast-phase direction of any nystagmus

Intention tremor

An intention tremor should have been detected as part of the examination of the limbs but can be retested here:

1. ask them to touch their nose with their forefinger, and then to touch your finger; ensure that the patient has to fully stretch their arm out to reach the target

2. test both sides
3. note whether they miss the target and whether a tremor emerges as their finger approaches the target
4. also test for impaired check by (1) asking the patient to hold their arms up like a boxer and to resist your pull; (2) pull against their biceps; (3) release suddenly, noting if their flexed arm pulls back in an exaggerated manner

Speech
Speech is usually evident from the initial examination, but ask them (1) to describe the room, looking for dysarthria or scanning speech and (2) to say 'Lah', 'Gah', 'But'.

Hypotonia
Take the patient's arms and legs in turn and check for tone if not already assessed.

Dysdiodochokinesia
Dysdiodochokinesia can be demonstrated:
1. ask the patient to clap one hand on top of the other, turning it from front to back each time
2. demonstrate this for them
3. note any slowed or poorly co-ordinated efforts
4. check their heel–shin co-ordination as described in Chapter 5 (see page 129)

Key findings
Each of the VANISHD symptoms or signs can occur with lesions in places other than the cerebellum, but a cerebellar lesion should still always be considered. Unilateral cerebellar lesions tend to produce ipsilateral signs, in contrast to cerebral lesions which produce contralateral signs. There are distinct 'cerebellar syndromes' comprising a constellation of these symptoms that point to a particular anatomical location of the lesion. These are summarised in **Table 6.1**. Cerebellar disease has many underlying causes, including developmental, hereditary and acquired (**Table 6.2**).

Syndrome	Location of lesion	Predominant clinical features
Rostral vermis syndrome	Anterior lobe/rostral vermis	Broad-based gait Truncal ataxia
Caudal vermis syndrome	Posterior or flocculonodular lobe	Vertigo Staggering gait Truncal ataxia Nystagmus
Hemispheric syndrome	Cerebellar hemisphere	Limb ataxia Intention tremor Dysmetria Dysarthria Dysdiodokokinesia

Table 6.1 Cerebellar syndromes. Lesions of the vermis tend to cause more truncal ataxia than limb ataxia, and fewer obvious limb signs. Lesions in the hemispheres cause a greater range of symptoms and include prominent limb signs ipsilateral to the lesion

Developmental or hereditary

Key causes include Arnold–Chiari and Dandy–Walker malformations and the hereditary ataxias.

Arnold–Chiari malformation

This is often asymptomatic or can present with headaches or nystagmus.

Dandy–Walker malformation

This may present with hydrocephalus or delayed development in childhood. Other features such as nystagmus commonly occur.

The hereditary ataxias

These include a large number of rare autosomal dominant and recessive conditions:

- the most common autosomal dominant conditions are the spinocerebellar ataxias, which are chronic, progressive

Type	Cause
Hereditary	Friedreich's ataxia Spinocerebellar ataxias Episodic ataxias Ataxia-telangectasia Leukodystrophies Urea cycle disorders Mitochondrial disorders
Developmental and/or structural	Dandy–Walker malformation Arnold–Chiari malformation
Vascular	Ischaemic stroke (usually posterior inferior cerebellar artery) Haemorrhagic stroke (can lead to hydrocephalus)
Neoplastic	Metastasis Astrocytoma Glioma Medulloblastoma Ependymoma Von Hippel–Lindau syndrome
Infective	Epstein–Barr virus Herpes simplex virus Abscess
Immune	Coeliac Multiple sclerosis Paraneoplastic syndrome
Toxins or drugs	Phenytoin Carbamazepine Sodium valproate Amiodarone Lithium Alcohol
Systemic disease	Liver disease Thyroid disease

Table 6.2 Causes of cerebellar signs or symptoms

conditions. There is usually a family history and genetic testing for mutations (which are usually CAG trinucleotide repeats) is available

- the most common autosomal recessive condition is Friedreich's ataxia. This is a chronic, progressive disease with onset between infancy and the twenties. There is often areflexia of the ankles, cardiomyopathy and diabetes in up to one-quarter of cases

Acquired

There are a wide range of acquired causes of cerebellar disease, including vascular, toxic, neoplastic, infective and immune-mediated pathologies.

Vascular

Posterior circulation syndrome ischaemic strokes commonly cause cerebellar signs (**Table 3.5**). Haemorrhage into the cerebellum accounts for 10% of intracerebral haemorrhage. This causes headache in addition to cerebellar symptoms and commonly causes decreased consciousness and may lead to life-threatening hydrocephalus.

Toxins

Alcohol is the most common toxic cause. Chronic overuse can lead to Wernicke's (ataxia, acute confusion, eye movement disorder) or Korsakoff's syndromes (a chronic amnesic state).

Benzodiazepines, phenytoin, carbamazepine, chemotherapeutic drugs and lithium are the more common drugs associated with dysarthria and ataxia.

Tumours

In children medulloblastomas, astrocytomas and ependymomas are relatively common primary tumours found in the cerebellum. In adults, cerebellar tumours are usually metastases. Paraneoplastic syndromes causing cerebellar syndromes are well described and are usually the result of small cell lung carcinoma or breast cancer.

What happens next?

The next step is to examine higher cortical function. Cerebellar syndromes require investigation with MRI as CT poorly visualises the posterior fossa.

Patients with cerebellar disease not readily explained by vascular causes or alcohol usually require careful and extensive investigation. Revisiting the family history is an ideal place to start and it may be helpful to actually see and examine family members.

6.6 System summary

A summary for examining for cerebellar disease is given in **Table 6.3**.

General observations	Inspect body and feet Palpate pulse, auscultate carotids Palpate abdomen
Vertigo	
Ataxia	Sitting Standing Walking
Nystagmus	Primary gaze Gaze evoked
Intention tremor	Reassess with finger–nose test Test for impaired check
Speech	Note any dysarthria or scanning speech
Hypotonia	Assess tone in limbs
Dysdiadochokinesia	Test alternating clapping
	Test heel–shin

Table 6.3 Cerebellar examination

Higher cortical function

7.1 Objectives

Examination of higher cortical function is less useful for fine localisation, but it is very helpful in determining the impact of a disease process on a patient's cognitive processes and for assessing its progression over time. Two commonly-used bedside tests of cognition are the Mini-Mental State Examination (MMSE) and the Revised Addenbrooke's Cognitive Examination (ACE-R). These test the five basic cognitive domains, (attention and orientation, language, visuoperceptual function and calculation, memory and executive function) which are discussed below.

The Mini-Mental State Examination

The MMSE is a widely-used and quick method to screen for cognitive dysfunction. This is often all that is needed in patients without significant cognitive impairment and provides an assessment of:

- orientation
- registration (immediate memory)
- short-term memory
- language

The UK National Institute for Health and Clinical Excellence (NICE) classifies the degree of cognitive impairment according to the MMSE score, as shown in **Table 7.1**.

The Revised Addenbrooke's Cognitive Examination

The ACE-R is a more in-depth procedure used for more detailed screening and to

> ## Clinical insight
>
> Bear in mind that patients vary greatly in their background, education and culture. A subtle decline in calculation skills in a mathematics professor is more significant than in someone who left school aged 15. Some cultural groups may find some of the testing unusual or be uncomfortable being asked such questions and their responses can be easily misinterpreted.
>
> Mood disorders or medications affecting the CNS also impact on a patient's performance in a cognitive assessment.

Score	Degree of cognitive impairment
25–30	Normal
21–24	Mild
10–20	Moderate
<10	Severe

Table 7.1 Cognitive impairment is graded according to the patient's score on the MMSE

monitor medium- to long-term changes in cognitive function. It is also more reliable at distinguishing between different subtypes of dementia, such as Alzheimer's disease, frontotemporal dementia and supranuclear palsy. It is freely available online.

7.2 Anatomy and physiology review

Cognitive processes depend upon many interconnected cortical and subcortical structures distributed throughout the brain. Bedside cognitive examinations are not designed to tease out precise anatomical regions; language function is the exception, and is discussed below.

A practical categorisation of higher cognitive functions is to divide them into five major domains:
1. attention and orientation
2. language
3. visuoperceptual function and calculation
4. memory
5. executive function

Attention and orientation
These functions are 'basic' to other cognitive functions: a basic level of attention and awareness is required for language, memory, etc. It relies on a distributed network of cerebral areas, including the mesial temporal lobes.

Language

Language is such a defining feature of our human nature that the complexity of neural computations that it requires is easily overlooked. Indeed, language is perhaps the most complex function of the most complex structure in the universe. In recent years a 'dual stream model' of language processing has emerged. This proposes that speech recognition depends on neural circuits in both:

- the superior temporal lobes (the ventral stream)
- the frontoparietal–temporal circuit in the left hemisphere in the majority of people (the dorsal stream)

Broca's area is a cortical area on the dominant (left in most people) inferior frontal gyrus. It is part of the dorsal stream in the above model.

Wernicke's area was historically considered to be a cortical area on the dominant superior temporal gyrus. In the dual stream model this area is part of the ventral stream and both hemispheres contribute to this aspect of speech (**Figure 7.1**).

Visuoperceptual function and calculation

This includes functions such as spatial organisation, praxis (planning) and calculations. The phenomenon of 'neglect' consists of a specific deficit in this domain. The underlying

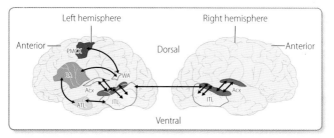

Figure 7.1 The dual stream model of language function. There is a bilateral ventral stream underlying speech recognition and a dorsal stream involved with speech production. BA, Broca's area; WA, Wernicke's area; PMcx, premotor cortex; Acx, auditory cortex; ATL, anterior temporal lobe; ITL, inferior temporal lobe.

brain regions involved remain controversial, but the parietal lobes and the parietal-temporal junction of the non-dominant hemisphere (usually the right) are important.

Memory

There are many types of memory. It is helpful to distinguish between short-term memory (or working memory) and long-term memory as they depend on different neuroanatomical substrates. It is also useful to be able to assess both verbal and visual memory. Again, the neuroanatomical regions involved in memory are legion; however, the hippocampus and other mesial temporal lobe structures are crucial for the formation of declarative memories and, in particular, working memory.

Executive function

This term refers to some of the 'higher' cortical functions such as abstraction, inhibition, planning and other social behaviours. The frontal lobes and basal ganglia appear crucial for such tasks.

7.3 Clinical features and pathophysiology

Attention and orientation

Deficits in attention and memory can be caused by a wide range of pathologies:

- delirium: general metabolic derangement (e.g. from infection, drugs, hypoxia) is likely to cause globally impaired neuronal function. Patients become disorientated in time and place and unable to attend to stimuli or interact normally. This tends to fluctuate
- dementia: attention and orientation are markedly abnormal in the dementias. However, this tends not to be associated with the fluctuating level of consciousness seen in delirium
- psychiatric disorders: depression can cause a so-called pseudo-dementia, largely due to reduced attention and concentration leading to poor functioning in other domains. Mania and other psychopathology can appear as impaired attention or orientation (e.g. flight of ideas, circumstantiality)

Language

Because of the complexity of language and the multitude of brain regions underlying its various aspects, it is possible to distinguish many different types of language deficits. Many of them are associated with specific anatomical regions.

Comprehension

Language comprehension appears to be bilaterally localised along the superior temporal gyrus. Deficits in language comprehension are particularly socially isolating.

Receptive aphasia is the inability to understand language and is also known as Wernicke's aphasia or posterior aphasia.

> **Clinical insight**
>
> Wernicke's aphasia: damage to Wernicke's area in the superior temporal gyrus can cause a type of aphasia known as Wernicke's or receptive aphasia. The patient appears unable to understand language (i.e. cannot follow instructions), but is easily able to generate words and sentences even if these are grammatically and semantically meaningless.

Reading

Dyslexia is a developmental reading disorder which is usually evident in early childhood. Alexia refers to the acquired inability to read in someone previously able to. It is often found along with dysphasias and is associated with frontal and parietal lesions.

Writing

An inability to write is called agraphia. This is usually seen in dominant parietal lobe lesions.

Speech

Deficits in speech include:
- **dysphonia**: patients with parkinsonism often display a slow, monotonous and quiet speech
- **dysarthria**: this is a deficit in speech articulation. There is no deficit in speech content. It may be caused by a lesion in the motor cortex, internal capsule, brainstem, cerebellum or cranial nerves

- **dysphasia**: receptive dysphasia is the inability to understand speech; expressive dysphasia is also known as Broca's or anterior aphasia and is impairment of the ability to generate speech not caused by a dysarthria. Depending on the location and extent of the lesion the problems can range from minor (e.g. a subtle nominal dysphasia with difficulty finding specific names of objects) to major (e.g. broken speech with great difficulty in communicating at all)

Significant language deficits are found in some of the dementias as well as in many types of localised lesions. Stroke is a major cause of language problems in Western populations. In these populations, a sudden onset expressive or receptive dysphasia strongly suggests a stroke or transient ischaemic attack.

Visuoperceptual function and calculation

Impaired visuoperceptual function and calculation manifests as:
- poor spatial organisation
- neglect
- impaired praxis
- problems with simple arithmetic and everyday tasks such as shopping

These tasks require a baseline level of attention and concentration and so can be impaired when other cognitive domains are primarily affected.

Testing this domain involves:
- drawing tasks
- copying multistep movements or procedures
- arithmetic

These can be impaired in most global encephalopathies, but in terms of dementias tend to be mildly impaired in Alzheimer's disease and more severely affected in corticobasal degeneration and dementia with Lewy bodies.

They are also commonly impaired in non-dominant hemisphere strokes, giving rise to the common features in these patients of neglect and dyspraxia.

Memory

The lateral temporal lobes are crucial sites for semantic memory processes. Memory can appear falsely impaired owing to poor concentration in depressive states. Alzheimer's disease, dementia with Lewy bodies and frontal–temporal dementia all exhibit profound memory deficits. Progressive supranuclear palsy is typically associated with well-preserved memory function, and can thereby be distinguished from other neurodegenerative processes.

Executive function

Deficits in executive functioning often cause substantial impairment in an individual's ability to work and to participate normally in social activities. Deficits in this domain may not be apparent on initial discussion or history taking. Basic tests of executive function examine:

- initiation
- abstraction
- set-shifting

Executive functioning tends to be affected in most degenerative cognitive processes. In many ways it defines a dementing process; however, it may be quite well preserved in mild cognitive impairment.

7.4 Bedside testing of cognitive domains

Objective

The purpose of this part of the examination is two-fold:

1. to perform a brief screen of the five basic cognitive domains
2. to elicit a number of cortical release signs or 'primitive reflexes'

The following approach assesses each of the five domains in turn. Some elements of it are in common with the ACE-R and

MMSE but it includes slightly more detailed assessment than either.

Approach
Firstly, ask the patient whether they are naturally left or right handed. Then tell the patient that you are going to test their memory and speech with some very simple questions that will get a bit more difficult.

Equipment
This stage of the examination requires paper, pen, a photograph and a newspaper.

Sequence
Examine cognitive function by domain:
- orientation
- attention
- language
- visuoperceptual function and calculation
- memory
- executive function
- cortical release signs (primitive reflexes)

Orientation
Ask the patient the:
- time (hour, day of week, month, year)
- place (ward, building, town, country)
- person (their name, age and date of birth)

Attention
Test attention by asking the patient to:
- recite the months of the year backwards
- spell WORLD backwards
- repeat back 7–9 sequentially longer numbers (a test of digit-span memory)

Language
Assess language function for:

- lack of comprehension (receptive dysphasia)
- poor articulation (dysarthria)
- problems expressing or word finding (expressive dysphasia)

> ### Clinical insight
>
> When testing a patient's ability to repeat a span of digits, remember to write down the numbers for yourself to check whether they are right!

To assess language, test the patient's abilities of:

- **conversation**: note the length, word choice, articulation and fluency of speech during the consultation
- **language function**: asking the patient to describe the picture in **Figure 7.2**
- **comprehension**: ask them the following: 'what colour are daffodils?' (yellow); 'what do we call a small seat without a back? (stool); 'touch your left cheek with your right thumb'
- **naming**: ask them to name a few objects close to hand (e.g. pen, belt, cup)

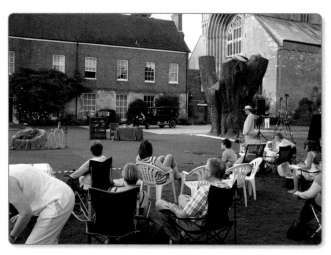

Figure 7.2 Picture used to assess language function. Patients should be asked to describe the photograph. Visual memory is then tested later by having the patient recall the picture.

- **repetition**: ask them to repeat: 'baby'; 'hippopotamus'; 'education'; a name and address (e.g. 'Peter Godfrey, 14 Woodbean Avenue, Durham') and tell them to try to remember it
- **writing**: ask them to write a short, sensible, sentence

Visuoperceptual function and calculation

Spatial organisation

Ask the patient to:

- draw a clock face, showing 'a quarter past six'
- copy the cube shown in **Figure 7.3**
- point to all the letter Bs in **Figure 7.4**
- name the fragmented letters in **Figure 7.5**

Neglect

Ask the patient to mark the exact mid-point of the horizontal line in **Figure 7.3**.

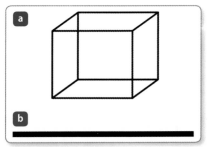

Figure 7.3 Visuospatial functions. (a) The cube is used to assess for a constructional dyspraxia. Ask the patient to copy this. They should include each side and each angle. (b) Ask the patient to bisect the line. In visual neglect they may place the midpoint off to one side

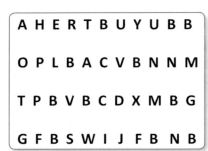

Figure 7.4 Ask the patient to count the number of letter Bs. Note any neglect. There are 11.

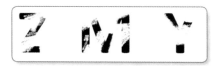

Figure 7.5 Ask the patient to name these letters. Z, M and Y are shown partially erased.

Praxis

Ask the patient to:
- copy a series of hand positions (**Figure 7.6**)
- demonstrate how they would 'hammer a nail in', 'brush their teeth', 'shave'
- if motor deficits allow, ask them to take off and/or put on their shirt or cardigan

Calculation

Ask the patient to perform some basic arithmetic.

Memory

To test the patient's memory, ask them:
- to recall the name and address from earlier
- to describe the picture you showed them
- 'who is the Prime Minister?'; 'what were the dates of the Second World War?'; and 'who was the US President assassinated in 1963?'
- to name a few famous people shown in a newspaper

Executive function

Proverbs

Have them explain the following proverbs:
- 'strike while the iron is hot'
- 'the apple never falls far from the tree'
- 'it is always darkest before the dawn'

Fluency

Have them name as many words as possible that begin with the letter C in 60 seconds.

Cortical release signs

Cortical release signs are generally insensitive, non-specific and not a formal part of any cognitive testing. However, when

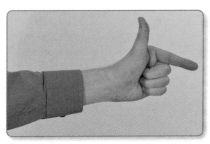

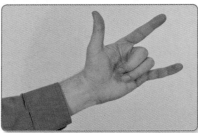

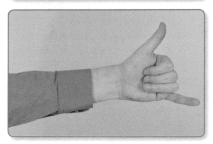

Figure 7.6 Testing praxis. Show the patient a number of hand positions to copy.

they occur in the clinical context of other frontal lobe signs or a history suggestive of cognitive impairment, they can be a useful pointer to frontal lobe dysfunction.

Grasp reflex

Stroke the patient's palm with your finger or end of the tendon hammer (**Figure 7.7**):

- normal: no grasp
- abnormal: hand involuntarily grips

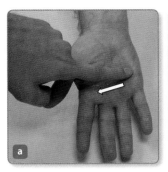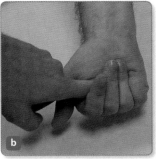

Figure 7.7 Grasp reflex: involuntary grasping of objects passing through the hand.

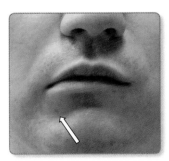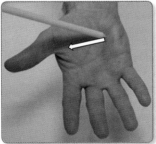

Figure 7.8 Palmomental reflex: a small ipsilateral contraction of the chin on stroking the palm.

Palmomental reflex

Stroke the thenar eminence with the end of the tendon hammer; observe the ipsilateral chin (**Figure 7.8**):
- normal: no chin movement
- abnormal: ipsilateral twitching of mentalis muscle

Pout reflex

Press firmly with your index finger on the patient's closed lips (**Figure 7.9**):
- normal: little resistance from lips

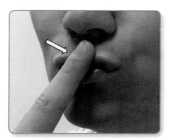

Figure 7.9 Pout reflex: on pressing the lips, the patient involuntarily forms a pout.

- abnormal: patient involuntarily pushes lips in a pouting or kissing movement

Key differential diagnoses

The value of assessing cognitive function lies in being able to recognise particular patterns of impairment across the different cognitive domains and interpreting these in light of the clinical context.

There are several common or important cognitive syndromes that will show deficits on bedside testing and that may be distinguished by the relative deficiencies in particular domains (**Table 7.2**).

> ### Clinical insight
>
> Around 15% of patients with mild cognitive impairment (MCI) go on to develop Alzheimer's disease each year. If a patient with MCI has abnormal levels of tau and phospho-tau proteins in their CSF, they have a much higher chance of developing Alzheimer's disease than if they have normal levels.

Mild cognitive impairment

Patients have subjective memory problems with some deficits on formal testing. Patients are able to function normally day to day with preserved general cognitive function.

Alzheimer's disease

This has slow onset and gradual progression of memory loss with impairment in other cognitive domains with time. Often, patients have language problems, apraxias or executive dysfunction.

Syndrome	Domains affected	Domains spared
Depression	All may be impaired, especially attention	–
Mild cognitive impairment	Mainly attention and short-term memory	Visuospatial, language, executive function may be normal initially
Alzheimer's disease	Marked attention, orientation and memory deficits. Language and visuospatial also affected	Eventually all cognitive domains become affected
Progressive supranuclear palsy	Executive function markedly impaired; memory	Language and visuospatial sometimes impaired
Dementia with Lewy bodies	Short-term memory and executive function	Most other domains spared until late
Frontotemporal dementia	Memory and executive function	Subtypes include patients with deficits primarily in language
Corticobasal degeneration	Executive function, language and visuospatial	Most domains eventually impaired
Multiple system atrophy	Memory and executive function	Most other domains spared until late

Table 7.2 Predominant deficits found in major subtypes of dementia

Vascular dementia

There is often executive dysfunction initially. There is also a characteristic stepwise pattern of abrupt declines in cognitive function in the presence of cerebrovascular disease.

Frontotemporal dementia

This can be either behavioural dominant or language dominant:

- behavioural-dominant patients show changes in personality and executive function

• language-dominant patients show expressive dysphasia
Both show memory impairment and characteristic preservation of visuospatial function.

Dementia with Lewy bodies
Patients have parkinsonism and cognitive dysfunction. There are characteristic fluctuations in attention and orientation, which may be mistaken for delirium. Visual and auditory hallucinations are common, as is a history of sleep disturbances.

Progressive supranuclear palsy
There is cognitive dysfunction in combination with signs and symptoms of supranuclear palsy, including vertical gaze palsy, pseudobulbar palsy and rigidity.

Corticobasal degeneration
Patients have cognitive dysfunction together with signs and symptoms of corticobasal degeneration, including asymmetrical rigidity. Cognitive impairment typically includes limb apraxia and neglect.

What happens next?
CT or MRI of the brain may be indicated. In dementias there will often be marked cortical atrophy, reflecting progressive loss of neuronal tissue. Specialised, radiolabelled neurotransmitter ligands or glucose imaging systems are used to assess the function of specific neurotransmitter systems (e.g. dopamine transmission in suspected Parkinson-plus syndromes) or whole-brain metabolic function (e.g. to look for characteristic patterns of cortical reduction in particular dementias). A MMSE or ACE-R test can be documented to help assess disease progression.

> **Clinical insight**
>
> There are two types of dementia: 'neat' or 'messy'. Although this hugely oversimplifies a complex spectrum, it highlights the way dementias tend to present: either with typical memory decline followed by other domains ('neat') or by unusual behavioural changes, usually reflecting early executive dysfunction ('messy').

7.5 System summary

A summary of higher cortical function examination is given in **Table 7.3**.

Orientation	Time, place, person
Attention	Months backwards
	WORLD backwards
	Digit span
Language	Note conversational speech
	Describe picture
	Comprehension: simple questions
	Name objects
	Repetition: 'baby', 'hippopotamus', name and address
	Write a short sentence
Visuospatial function and calculation	Clock face showing a specified time
	Copy cube
	Point to the letter Bs
	Name fragmented letters
	Neglect: line bisect
	Praxis: copy hand positions, pantomime actions, dressing
	Basic arithmetic
Memory Executive function Cortical release signs	Recall name and address from above
	Describe picture from above
	Questions: Prime Minister, Second World War, US President assassination
	Famous faces from a newspaper
	Proverbs
	Fluency: words beginning with C
	Grasp
	Palmomental
	Pout

Table 7.3 Summary of higher cortical function assessment

Autonomic nervous system

The autonomic nervous system (ANS) comprises the sympathetic and parasympathetic divisions in a diffuse network of central and peripheral connections that mediate homeostatic control of much of the body's 'vegetative functions'. The sympathetic and parasympathetic divisions generally act antagonistically to allow fine control over functions such as heart rate, blood pressure, respiration and a host of other core physiological functions.

8.1 Objectives

Both central nervous system (CNS) and peripheral nervous system lesions can affect the ANS. Often, the dysfunction is subtle and difficult to detect clinically owing to the large moment-to-moment and interindividual variation in many of the affected physiological parameters. However, it is essential to be aware of some simple bedside tests that can help in assessing the ANS.

The process explained in this chapter does not need to be carried out routinely in every patient; rather, it is required only in those with known neurological disease likely to involve the ANS or in those with relevant symptoms or signs from the history and remainder of the examination.

8.2 Anatomy and physiology review

The specific effects of the autonomic nervous system on selected organ systems are shown in **Table 8.1** and **Figure 8.1**. **Figure 8.2** shows the relation of the sympathetic chain and spinal cord.

The sympathetic and parasympathetic pathways both comprise preganglionic and postganglionic neurons:

- the preganglionic neurons have their cell bodies in the CNS and project to the postganglionic neurons
- the postganglionic neurons are located outside the CNS and mediate the effects on target organs

Target organ	Sympathetic stimulation (adrenergic)	Parasympathetic stimulation (muscarinic)
Eye: pupillary dilator	α_1 dilates pupil	M3 contracts pupil
Eye: ciliary muscle	β_2 relaxes	M3 contracts
Mouth	Stimulates thick saliva	Stimulates watery saliva
Gastrointestinal tract (motility)	Decreases	Increases
Lungs	β_2 relaxes bronchioles	M3 contracts bronchioles
Heart	Increases rate, contractility	Decreases rate, contractility
Vascular smooth muscle	α_1 constricts, β_2 relaxes	M3 relaxes
Arteries to skin	α_1 constricts	–
Bladder detrusor muscle	β_2 relaxes	M3 contracts
Urethral sphincters	α_1 contracts	M3 relaxes

Table 8.1 Major functions of the autonomic nervous system. α, alpha-adrenergic receptors. β, beta-adrenergic receptors; M3, muscarinic receptors

Clinical insight

Spinal cord lesions at T6 or above can lead to the syndrome of autonomic dysreflexia, characterised by life-threatening hypertensive crises. Peripheral noxious sensory stimulation (e.g. urinary retention) triggers an insufficiently-opposed sympathetic reflex in the spinal cord below the lesion, leading to marked systemic hypertension. Normally, descending inhibitory responses reduce this sympathetic storm, but with a cord lesion at T6 the descending inhibition cannot reach the thoracic cord to inhibit the storm. It does, however, reach the cervical and upper thoracic cord where it leads to flushing, sweating and dilation of the pupils.

Sympathetic nervous system

The sympathetic pathways:

- have postganglionic neurons mostly found in the sympathetic chain
- outflow emerges from spinal cord levels T1–L2 (thoracolumbar)
- broadly act in the 'fight or flight' response to increase efficient skeletal muscle energy supply, oxygen exchange, heart rate, etc.

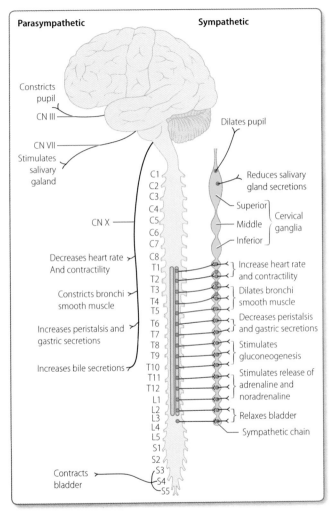

Figure 8.1 Summary of major functions of the sympathetic and parasympathetic components of the autonomic nervous system. The parasympathetic supply originates from the cranial nerves and caudal spinal cord. The sympathetic supply is derived mainly from the thoracic spinal cord and the sympathetic chain.

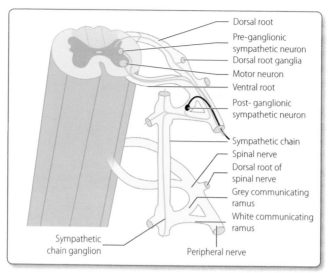

Figure 8.2 The sympathetic chain. Preganglionic sympathetic neurons send axons through the ventral root, spinal nerve and white communicating ramus to the sympathetic chain ganglia. Here the axons ascend and descend, project to target organ postganglionic neurons and also synapse locally on postganglionic sympathetic neurons within the ganglia. These send axons via the grey communicating ramus to join the peripheral nerve.

Parasympathetic nervous system

The parasympathetic pathways:

- have postganglionic neurons mostly found near or in their target organs
- outflow emerges from CN III, VII, X and S2–4 (craniosacral)
- broadly act to 'rest and digest': promote blood flow to the gastrointestinal tract and to oppose the sympathetic division

8.3 Clinical features and pathophysiology

Some important abnormal findings to be aware of include:

- **livido reticularis**: dusky cyanosis of the skin caused by swollen venules producing a characteristic blue lacy pattern. This has a wide differential diagnosis but may indicate dysfunction of control of the blood vessels

- **cold peripheries**: wide differential diagnosis, but may indicate chronic sympathetic denervation (which leads to upregulated receptors and chronic increased constriction in response to circulating catecholamines)
- **warm peripheries**: wide differential diagnosis, but a warm, red extremity may indicate an acute loss of sympathetic tone
- **anhidrosis** (lack of sweating): indicates a sympathetic lesion in the supply to the affected area
- **blood pressure**: this normally increases at least 10 mmHg on sustained handgrip. Less than this may indicate a central or peripheral sympathetic lesion
- **postural hypotension**:
  - drop of 20–30 mmHg systolic blood pressure (BP) on standing is abnormal
  - the normal small drop then small rise in diastolic BP is mediated by the IXth cranial nerve sensing a drop in BP at the carotid sinus and causing a compensatory increase in heart rate
  - failure of this reflex indicates sympathetic or parasympathetic dysfunction from a wide range of causes
- **heart rate variability**: the heart rate is a reflection of the fine balance between sympathetic and parasympathetic interplay. The following abnormalities may indicate an ANS lesion:
  - resting tachycardia (underactive parasympathetic)
  - loss of postural increase in heart rate (HR) (should increase by at least 10 bpm on standing)
  - no change in HR with the Valsalva manoeuvre (should increase during, and then slow after, Valsalva)
- **skin erythema**: skin blanching or erythema following mechanical pressure may be lost in peripheral lesions of the sympathetic system, or heightened in complex regional pain syndrome or below a spinal cord lesion
- **bladder**:
  - **urgency**: may be from frontal lobe lesions, chronic spinal cord lesions, overflow from peripheral neurogenic bladder (e.g. cauda equina syndrome)

- **retention**: may be from acute spinal cord lesions or from peripheral neurogenic bladder
- **bowel**: reduced anal tone or decreased perianal sensation (saddle anaesthesia) suggests a cauda equina lesion

8.4 History

Objective
The objective of the history is to elicit specific details relevant to autonomic dysfunction. These may have been missed because the patient fails to think they are significant or the doctor does not think to ask.

Approach
Tell the patient that you need to ask some questions relating to how the brain and nerves control some bodily functions.

Sequence
Work through the major functions of the ANS, checking for important symptoms of dysfunction. Key questions are:
1. 'any faint spells? What about on standing/coughing/straining/eating?'
2. 'any changes to your skin?'
3. 'do you get hot or sweaty flushes?'
4. 'any change in your bladder function? Any incontinence? Are you finding it more difficult to pass urine?'
5. 'are your bowels moving normally?'
6. 'can you feel it when you wipe after a bowel motion?'
7. 'any problems during sexual intercourse?' [in men, clarify whether there is failure of erection (parasympathetic) or failure of ejaculation (sympathetic)]
8. 'what medications are you taking?'

8.5 Bedside examination and tests

Objective
The purpose of this stage of the examination is to identify any major autonomic dysfunction. There is substantial interindividual variation in the parameters assessed, making these tests

somewhat difficult to interpret. However, they are nonetheless useful bedside tests.

Approach

Tell the patient you need to monitor their heart rate and blood pressure while they perform a few minor acts including lying, standing, straining and squeezing a ball.

Equipment

This requires an ECG machine, BP cuff and extra sphygmomanometer, and a pen torch.

Sequence

Follow the sequence:

1. look at the skin
2. feel the skin (temperature, oedema, etc.)
3. examine the pupils
4. attach the ECG machine and record the following: (a) lying pulse and BP; (b) standing pulse (initially and at 2–3 minutes) and BP (at 2–3 minutes); (c) heart rate variability during deep breathing (compare shortest and longest RR interval over 10 deep breaths); and (d) heart rate variability during Valsalva
5. ask the patient to squeeze the spare sphygmomanometer continuously and measure the BP at 2 minutes

> ### Clinical insight
>
> Back pain and urinary incontinence/retention is often assumed to be caused by cauda equina syndrome until proven otherwise. This may be a safe way to approach such patients but do not forget to take a proper history and examination in your haste. Renal tract pathology (e.g. pyelonephritis with back pain and dysuria) is often mistaken for cauda equina syndrome. Even patients in obvious septic shock have been treated as such. Take a thorough account of any change in bladder function, examine anal tone yourself and properly assess for perianal sensation.

Key findings

These include:

- **pupil abnormalities**: see Chapter 3 (see page 61)
- **postural hypotension/loss of postural tachycardia**: this has many causes and is often multifactorial, especially in

the elderly. It may indicate a sympathetic lesion (e.g. Guillain–Barré syndrome, diabetic neuropathy or multisystems atrophy)

- **skin**: cold peripheries indicate a chronic sympathetic lesion; warm, red peripheries or affecting a single limb indicate acute loss of sympathetic tone. This can result from complex regional pain syndrome or an acute sympathetic lesion from any cause (e.g. Guillain–Barré syndrome, brachial plexopathy)
- **Valsalva manoeuvre**: lack of an increase in heart rate during the manoeuvre indicates a sympathetic lesion; lack of a decrease in heart rate after the manoeuvre indicated a parasympathetic lesion
- **peripheral neurogenic bladder**: this will have the following features:
  - typically painless urinary retention
  - with or without overflow incontinence
  - there may be other signs of cauda equina syndrome such as faecal incontinence, saddle anaesthesia, radicular pain in the legs and weakness of ankle dorsiflexion
  - causes include cauda equina syndrome and diabetic neuropathy
- **spinal cord bladder**: this will have the following features:
  - acute: urinary retention and overflow
  - chronic: small volumes of involuntary voiding
- **cortical bladder**: control of voiding is normally regulated via the cingulate gyrus and paracentral gyrus. Lesions here (stroke, demyelination, hydrocephalus) can cause unawareness of a distended bladder with overflow urination

Clinical insight

Conditions commonly showing dysfunction of the autonomic nervous system include:

- diabetes mellitus
- third nerve palsy
- spinal cord injury
- multiple systems atrophy
- trigeminal autonomic cephalgia

What happens next?

A bedside bladder scanner is useful to detect any retention and determine whether incontinence is from overflow. CT or MRI of the brain and spinal cord may be indicated depending on the history and examination findings.

More detailed assessment of urinary dysfunction is possible via urodynamics and a urology referral should be made if there is no clear cause.

8.6 System summary

A summary of examination of the autonomic nervous system is shown in **Table 8.2**.

History	Bladder, bowels, syncope, skin, sweating, sensation, sex, medications
Inspection	Skin
	Pupils
Bedside tests	Lying and standing pulse and blood pressure
	Heart rate variability (lying, standing, breathing, Valsalva, hand grip).

Table 8.2 Summary of assessment of the autonomic nervous system

Examining the stroke patient

Every junior doctor should be competent in the recognition, initial assessment and management of acute stroke. It is a common and serious condition that requires immediate management decision-making.

Despite the need for a speedy assessment, the history remains crucial and must be carried out properly and appropriate collateral history sought where needed. Most hospitals now have an acute stroke service and they should be contacted early for discussion of appropriate investigations and management.

9.1 Objectives

Assessing the patient with acute onset of focal neurological symptoms requires a balance between speed and thoroughness to ensure:

- symptoms and signs are confirmed
- stroke risk factors are identified
- the lesion is broadly localised
- suitability for thrombolysis is established

9.2 Anatomy and physiology review

Many are apprehensive of assessing the stroke patient as they are convinced a detailed knowledge of neuroanatomy and arterial territories is required. Although this helps with fine localisation and in rarer presentations, only a broad knowledge is required.

The widespread implementation of the Oxford classification system allows a pragmatic approach to classifying stroke in the acute setting. This classification groups strokes into four main categories based on the clinical features. This allows broad localisation of pathology to the:

- carotid arteries
- vertebrobasilar arterial system

Guiding principles

The stroke assessment need to be:
- **Speedy,** to allow for thrombolysis
- **Specific,** to identify the stroke syndrome
- **Safe,** to identify stroke mimics needing urgent treatment

A well-rehearsed stroke exam, familiarity with the major stroke syndromes and always being mindful of stroke mimics are the secrets to a successful stroke assessment.

- deep perforating arteries
- superficial cortical vessels

These broad divisions are helpful in directing immediate and long-term investigations and management and inform the prognosis. The classification is shown in **Table 9.1**.

The Oxford system is based on clinical features but these correlate with typical blood vessel dysfunction. Thus, disturbances in blood flow in the carotid arteries (the

Syndrome	Features
Total anterior circulation syndrome	All of: Motor or sensory deficit* Hemianopia Higher cortical dysfunction
Partial anterior circulation syndrome	Two of: Motor or sensory deficit Hemianopia Higher cortical dysfunction
Lacunar syndrome	One of: Pure motor deficit* Pure sensory deficit* Sensorimotor deficit* Ataxic hemiparesis Without any of: Higher cortical dysfunction Posterior circulation syndrome symptoms
Posterior circulation syndrome	Any of: Isolated homonymous hemianopia Bilateral motor or sensory deficit Brainstem signs Cerebellar signs

Table 9.1 The Oxford stroke classification system. *Affecting face, arm and leg.

anterior circulation) lead to TACS or PACS, while disturbances to flow in the vertebrobasilar vessels (the posterior circulation) leads to POCS. **Figure 9.1** illustrates the division of the anterior and posterior circulations. **Figure 9.2** shows the circle of Willis and major arteries.

9.3 Clinical features and pathophysiology

Stroke is defined as the sudden onset of focal neurological symptoms which localise to a vascular territory or territories, lasting more than 24 hours.

Transient ischaemic attacks (TIAs) last less than 24 hours by definition but most last less than a few hours. The risk of a further stroke after a TIA is high (8–12% 7-day risk; 18% 30-day risk) and should therefore be investigated promptly.

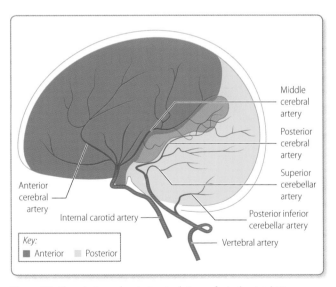

Figure 9.1 The anterior and posterior circulations refer to the circulation derived from the internal carotid arteries (anterior; green) and the vertebrobasilar arteries (posterior; yellow)

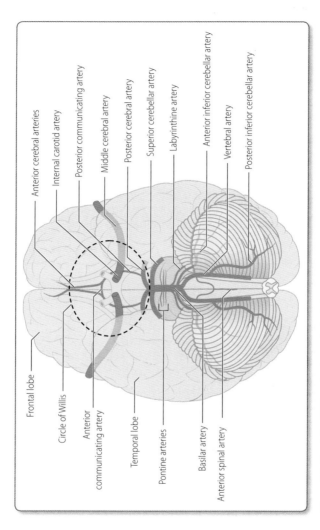

Figure 9.2 The circle of Willis and major cerebral arteries.

There are many causes, however:

- most strokes are ischaemic (80%): atherothromboembolism, cardioembolism and small vessel disease constitute the majority of causes of ischaemic stroke
- haemorrhagic stroke is sufficiently common that empirical treatment of suspected stroke without brain imaging is unsafe

Major risk factors for ischaemic stroke are shown in **Table 9.2**. Smoking and diabetes also double the risk.

The hallmark of neurological problems caused by stroke is the sudden loss of neurological function. Loss of vision, speech problems, numbness and weakness are typical whereas positive phenomena such as visual flashes or paraesthesia are unusual. The Oxford classification describes four syndromes:

- lacunar syndrome
- partial anterior circulation syndrome
- total anterior circulation syndrome
- posterior circulation syndrome

Lacunar syndrome

A lacunar infarct occurs in the deep penetrating arteries of the thalamus, corona radiata or internal capsule. Lacunar syndrome consists of:

> ## Guiding principles
>
> Anterior circulation strokes result from pathologies affecting the carotid artery and its branches:
>
> - atherosclerosis of carotid artery
> - small vessel disease
> - cardiac embolism
>
> Posterior circulation strokes result from pathologies affecting the vertebral artery and its branches:
>
> - cardiac embolism
> - atheroslcerosis of vertebral artery
> - dissection of artery

Risk factor	Relative risk
Hypertension (systolic over 160)	7
Age (over 75)	5
Atrial fibrillation	5
Previous transient ischaemic attack/stroke	5
Ischaemic heart disease	3

Table 9.2 Major risk factors for ischaemic stroke

- pure motor deficit
- pure sensory deficit
- or both
- it must involve two or more of the face, arm and leg
- no other new neurological symptoms are present

Partial anterior circulation syndrome

A partial anterior circulation syndrome (PACS) occurs when part of the anterior circulation (the vasculature derived from the internal carotid arteries) is occluded. It differs from a total anterior circulation syndrome (TACS) in the extent of brain that is ischaemic and is usually from a more distal occlusion than a TACS. It consists of two of the following:

- motor or sensory deficit [from occlusion of the middle branch of the middle cerebral artery (MCA)]
- higher cortical dysfunction (from occlusion of the middle or anterior branch of the MCA)
- hemianopia (from occlusion of the posterior branch of the MCA).

Total anterior circulation syndrome

A TACS occurs when the whole of the anterior circulation is occluded. There is a 'full house' of symptoms:

- motor deficit
- sensory deficit
- homonymous hemianopia
- higher cortical dysfunction

Posterior circulation syndrome

A posterior circulation syndrome (POCS) is caused by an infarct in the territory supplied by the arteries derived from the vertebral and basilar arteries. This presents with:

- an isolated hemianopia
- brainstem signs (e.g. cranial nerve palsies)
- cerebellar ataxia

The spectrum of clinical findings can be wide and confusing when there is brainstem involvement as there are many motor, sensory and cranial nerve tracts and nuclei close together in this region (see Figure 3.2 and Table 3.5).

Hemispheric dominance

The left hemisphere is dominant and houses language function in 95% of right-handed people and 70% of left-handed people. Along

with the expected weakness, hemianopia, etc. on the contralateral side of the body, a stroke in each hemisphere usually results in quite typical higher cortical dysfunction (**Table 9.3**).

9.4 Stroke: history

Objective

The purpose of this examination is to establish the range of symptoms, identify the timing of onset as accurately as possible, identify risk factors, identify any clear cause, identify other comorbidities and determine suitability for thrombolysis.

Approach

Patients are often dysphasic, disorientated or otherwise unable to give a reliable history. It is imperative to obtain a collateral history from family or eye witnesses in order to establish clearly the timing of onset and any contraindications to thrombolysis.

Telephone family members or witnesses if needed and, if there is time (e.g. while waiting for a referral to arrive in the emergency department), contact their relevant healthcare providers such as GP or other physician to establish premorbid state, comorbidities or recent interventions. However, do not delay the rest of the assessment for this.

	Dominant (usually left)	Non-dominant (usually right)
Clinical features	Aphasia, poor right conjugate gaze, difficulty reading, writing or calculating	Extinction, neglect, poor left conjugate gaze, spatial disorientation
Patient insight	Usually present	Usually absent

Table 9.3 Clinical features of dominant and non-dominant hemisphere strokes

Sequence

Key information to establish in a stoke history is:

1. the time of onset:
   - if the patient is unable to clarify, this must be assumed to be the time last known to be well
   - for patients waking up with stroke symptoms this must be assumed to be when they went to sleep
2. which symptoms are present:
   - weakness, numbness, speech problems, visual disturbance, swallowing problems, ataxia, vertigo
3. whether symptoms are improving, worsening or are static
4. risk factors present:
   - age
   - hypertension
   - diabetes
   - smoking
   - atrial fibrillation
   - ischaemic heart disease or peripheral vascular disease
   - hyperlipidaemia
   - alcohol
   - family history
5. premorbid state and comorbidities:
   - level of independence
   - employment
   - social activities
   - heart disease
   - gastrointestinal (GI) disease, especially liver disease and upper or lower GI bleeding
   - respiratory disease
   - neurological disease, including migraine
6. medication history:
   - full drug history, including recreational drugs
   - particularly use of antiplatelet drugs or anticoagulation
   - use of insulin or antihyperglycaemic drugs
7. contraindications to thrombolysis (see **Table 9.4**)

Thrombolysis contraindications	
Presentation	Onset unclear or more than 3.5 hours ago
	Seizure since onset
	Invasive/surgical procedure in previous 3 weeks
	Cardiopulmonary resuscitation
	Pregnancy
	Symptoms minor or improving
	Significant premorbid dependence.
Bleeding disorder	Previous intracranial bleeding
	Active bleeding
	Active peptic ulcer or gastrointestinal bleeding;
	Current anticoagulation use
Cranial disorders	Stroke in the preceding 3 months
	Head or facial trauma in the preceding 3 months
	Structural cerebrovascular disease
Cardiovascular	Aortic dissection
	Severe hypertension
	Diabetic retinopathy

Table 9.4 Contraindications to thrombolytic therapy

Key differential diagnoses

The history may suggest a typical TACS, PACS, POCS or lacunar syndrome. Other conditions may closely mimic ischaemic stroke and include:

- haemorrhagic stroke: there is no absolute way to differentiate but this more commonly presents with headache than ischaemic stroke
- hypoglycaemia can occur in patients with known diabetes on medical therapy
- complicated migraine: patients may have atypical features for stroke, such as positive visual phenomena or paraesthesia, and a history of migraines

- hyper or hypocalcaemia
- sepsis, especially in elderly, may cause focal neurological symptoms

What happens next?
Perform a modified (stroke) neurological examination and a general examination.

9.5 Stroke: neurological examination

Objective
The aim of the stroke neurological examination is to identify neurological signs in order to classify the stroke syndrome, broadly localise the lesion and allow immediate management decision-making.

Approach
This is essentially a general neurological examination aimed at eliciting the major signs required to classify the syndrome.

Equipment
This requires a tendon hammer, pen torch, hat pin, examination pin and tuning fork.

Sequence
To perform a focused stroke examination:
1. assess the Glasgow Coma Scale score (see Table 10.1)
2. orientation: ask the month and the patient's age
3. commands: ask the patient to open and close their eyes, then grip and release with their non-paretic hand
4. assess cranial nerves III, IV, VI: note any cranial nerve or gaze palsy
5. assess for visual defects: tested with the hat pin, confrontation or visual threat as appropriate
   - hemianopia
   - visual neglect
   - visual extinction

6. assess for weakness: face, arms, legs
7. limb ataxia: test finger–nose pointing and heel–shin co-ordination
8. sensation: test pin-prick sensation or withdrawal to pain
   - face
   - arms
   - legs
   - sensory extinction or neglect
   - further assess vibration sense when there is clinical suspicion of a brainstem lesion
9. language: ask the patient to describe what you are wearing, name items and read a sentence
10. dysarthria: ask the patient to repeat words
11. test the limb and plantar reflexes

Key differential diagnoses

It should be possible to identify the stroke syndrome and classify it within the Oxford classification or localise it further. Hypoglycaemia must be excluded in all patients as it can cause sudden onset focal neurological deficits. Migraine can uncommonly cause unusual transient neurological deficits and can mimic stroke. It is not always possible to clinically differentiate this from true stroke.

What happens next?

Next, perform a brief general examination.

9.6 Stroke: general examination

Objective

This examination is used to identify evidence of any predisposing factors, extent of coexistent disease and complications of stroke. These include:

- evidence of stroke risk factors (**Table 9.2**)
- evidence of complications of stroke such as aspiration pneumonia
- evidence of contraindications to thrombolysis (retinopathy, peptic ulcer, GI bleeding)

Equipment

This requires a stethoscope and an ophthalmoscope.

Sequence

The key body system areas to examine are cardiovascular, respiratory and gastrointestinal.

Cardiovascular

Assess the following:

- heart rate and rhythm (e.g. atrial fibrillation)
- murmurs (e.g. septic emboli from endocarditis)
- blood pressure (hyper- or hypotension, aortic dissection)
- bruits (poor correlation with carotid artery atheroma)
- fundoscopy (diabetic or hypertensive retinopathy)
- peripheral pulses (vascular disease)

Respiratory

Assess the following:

- respiratory rate (sepsis, pneumonia)
- focal chest signs (aspiration)

Gastrointestinal

Assess the following:

- peripheral stigmata of liver disease
- abdominal tenderness may reflect peptic ulcer disease or mesenteric ischaemia
- per rectum bleeding

What happens next?

Obtain an ECG and a blood glucose reading. Discuss the patient with the acute stroke team regarding their suitability for thrombolysis and further management. If thrombolysis is being considered, an immediate CT brain scan is required to exclude haemorrhage.

CT

A CT scan should be performed quickly to exclude haemorrhage. Note that a CT may be normal early on or in posterior circulation syndrome infarcts. MRI is far more sensitive and is indicated if the CT is normal or in posterior circulation syndromes. However, this takes longer than CT and is not usually available in the acute setting.

An acute ischaemic stroke may appear normal or it may be evident as:

- **sulci effacement**: cortical sulci lose definition owing to subtle oedema

> ## Clinical insight
>
> Decreasing consciousness in the first few days following a stroke can be the first sign of a neurosurgical emergency:
>
> - malignant middle cerebral artery syndrome results from raised intracranial pressure caused by progressive swelling of a large hemispheric stroke. It requires urgent decompressive craniectomy
> - hydrocephalus results from posterior fossa strokes with progressive swelling and obstruction of CSF flow. It requires decompressive craniectomy or an extra-ventricular drain

- **loss of grey–white differentiation**: oedema can cause subtle loss of distinction between grey and white matter, especially the lentiform nucleus of the basal ganglia and the cortical ribbon of the insular cortex
- **dense middle cerebral artery** (MCA): an occluded MCA can appear hyperdense on CT, as can an occluded basilar artery

9.7 Acute stroke treatments

Acute ischaemic stroke is treated with IV thrombolytics (e.g. alteplase) or intra-arterial clot retrieval if identified early enough.

Treatment of haemorrhagic stroke is different. It requires aneurysmal coiling or clipping (in cases of SAH), surgical removal of the haemorrhage, or surgical treatment of raised intracranial pressure from hydrocephalus.

Ischaemic stroke

Acute ischaemic stroke is treated with either IV thrombolytics or clot retrieval. For both options, earlier treatment provides greater benefits.

IV thrombolysis

IV thrombolysis (alteplase) is used to treat acute ischaemic stroke within 3.5 hours of onset:

- it reduces longer-term disability, which is often seen in both treated and untreated patients
- the degree of benefit decreases with time from onset, so that even though 3.5 hours is seen as the time limit the benefit at this stage is marginal

The decision to thrombolyse should be made by an experienced stroke consultant who can weigh the risks and benefits for the individual patient.

The risks of thrombolysis (gastrointestinal and intracranial haemorrhage) must be explained to the patient or next of kin by a physician experienced with its use.

Clot retrieval and thrombectomy

The physical removal of an acutely formed arterial clot is known as clot retrieval or thrombectomy. It is beneficial within 8 hours in patients with large MCA clots that have not resolved following IV thrombolytic administration. It is performed by an experienced interventional neuroradiologist using an intra-arterial catheter and X-ray-guided imaging. Its use is restricted to centres that can provide:

- readily accessible arterial imaging (e.g. CT angiography) to confirm the clot position
- experienced interventional neuroradiologists
- appropriate post-procedural monitoring (e.g. intensive care)

Surgical treatments

A number of surgical treatments can be considered for treating some types of stroke or their complications:

- SAH from an aneurysm requires coiling or clipping, if possible (see below)
- some patients with intracerebral haematomas benefit from their surgical removal
- decompression of a large, swollen hemisphere or the posterior fossa can be life-saving in large MCA territory strokes or cerebellar strokes
- CSF diversion can be helpful in acute hydrocephalus

Aneurysmal coiling or clipping

Patients who survive the initial haemorrhage from a ruptured cerebral berry (narrow-necked) aneurysm

> ### Clinical insight
>
> Basilar artery thrombosis may also benefit from thrombectomy if IV thrombolytics fail to restore perfusion.

will have the remaining aneurysm treated via an interventional neuroradiological procedure, called endovascular coiling, to prevent re-bleeding. This is done within a few days, preferably within 24 h. If the aneurysm is awkwardly shaped then open surgery with clipping of the aneurysm may be required.

Haematoma evacuation

Patients with superficial, large haematomas causing significant mass effect or hydrocephalus may benefit from having the haematoma surgically removed. Routine removal of smaller or deep haematomas does not improve outcome.

Decompression

Patients with large MCA territory infarcts often experience a malignant cycle of oedema, in which progressively worsening impairment of blood supply and further oedema lead to uncontrolled swelling of the affected hemisphere. If untreated this often leads to brain herniation and death. Removing the overlying skull decompresses the affected tissue and allows it to swell out through the skull defect rather than compressing the brainstem, and can be life-saving. It does not improve the prognosis of the underlying stroke.

Haemorrhage or infarct in the posterior fossa can also lead to uncontrolled swelling in this area, leading to blockage of the CSF flow and acute hydrocephalus. Decompression of the posterior fossa in this situation can also be life-saving.

CSF diversion

Patients with acute hydrocephalus following a stroke, from either oedema or blood blocking CSF flow, may benefit from insertion of an extraventricular drain to divert CSF flow and reduce intracranial pressure. When the acute phase has resolved this is then removed.

9.8 System summary

Table 9.5 summarises the examination of a stroke patient.

History	Time of onset, symptoms, progression, risk factors, premorbid disease, medications, contraindications to thrombolysis
Neurological assessment	Glasgow Coma Scale score
	Orientation
	Commands
	CN III, IV, VI
	Visual defects
	Weakness
	Limb ataxia
	Sensation
	Language
	Dysarthria
	Reflexes
General examination	
Bedside investigations (ECG blood glucose)	
Discussion with acute stroke team	
CT or MRI brain scan	

Table 9.5 Summary of the examination of a stroke patient

Examining the coma patient

10.1 Objectives

The key objectives when examining a person in a coma are to assess the level of consciousness, localise the lesion and detect any signs of the aetiology. This chapter assumes that the patient has been resuscitated following standard advanced life support or advanced trauma life support procedures and is otherwise stable.

10.2 Anatomy and physiology review

Normal consciousness requires an intact cerebral cortex and ascending brainstem reticular activating system (RAS). The RAS includes the midbrain reticular formation, the tegmentum and the thalamus. Cholinergic and adrenergic neurons ascend from these nuclei and form extensive connections with the thalamus, which in turn forms diffuse thalamocortical connections.

10.3 Clinical features and pathophysiology

Lesion localisation in unconscious patients can be difficult. However, there are a few general principles that allow identification of diffuse, hemispheric or brainstem lesions.

Brainstem lesions

Damage to the brainstem can cause decreased consciousness along with specific more focal symptoms. The presence of otherwise normal brainstem function (e.g. reflexes) therefore points towards a diffuse or cortical cause of decreased consciousness.

Signs indicating brainstem involvement include the following.

Eyes

The position of the eye and the presence of abnormal spontaneous movements can help localise a lesion.

Resting eye position

There are a number of key findings:

- in a gaze paresis from a **pontine lesion** the patient will be looking towards a hemiparesis and away from the lesion
- in a gaze paresis from a **hemisphere lesion** the patient will be looking away from a hemiparesis and towards the lesion. Dysfunction of the frontal eye fields removes the normal tonic drive of eyes, thereby allowing the intact hemisphere to draw the eyes towards it

> ## Clinical insight
>
> Remember **CAP** to help you localise a lesion in relation to a hemiparesis: In **C**ortical lesions the eyes look **A**way from the **P**aretic limb. Therefore, look at the patient: if they have a gaze paresis looking away from the paretic limb, the lesion must be in the cortex in the contralateral hemisphere; if they are looking towards the limb, it is a brainstem lesion.

- downgaze suggests a dorsal **midbrain** or **thalamic lesion**, or CN III, IV or VI lesions. It can also be caused by raised intracranial pressure: a so-called 'false localising sign'

Spontaneous eye movements

There are a number of key findings:

- slow roving horizontal eye movements suggest intact pontine and midbrain circuits and imply cortical damage
- ocular bobbing (downward jerking of eyes) suggests loss of horizontal gaze mechanisms at the base of the pons

Pupils

Pupils can be:

- **bilateral pin-point**: small, unreactive pupils suggest a pontine lesion or opiates
- **bilateral mid-position**: 4–6 mm, unreactive pupils suggest a midbrain lesion
- **bilateral dilated**: large, unreactive dilated pupils suggest anticholinergic poisoning or a preterminal stage of herniation

- **unilateral dilated**: suggests CN III palsy, e.g. from uncal herniation
- **normal**: metabolic causes other than opiate or anticholinergic poisoning generally do not affect the pupils

> ## Clinical insight
>
> Remember the localisation of abnormal pupils as: Pin-Point Pupils are Pontine or oPiate; Mid-position pupils are Midbrain.

Ocular reflexes

These are used when there are no spontaneous eye movements to help determine whether the brainstem is intact. There are two main reflexes:

- oculocephalic reflex (doll's eyes reflex)
  - 'positive' if intact; the patient's eyes will show slow conjugate deviation to the contralateral side when their head is turned (eyes appear to maintain fixation on a point)
  - 'negative' suggests brainstem involvement
- oculovestibular reflex (caloric testing)
  - this is performed if the oculocephalic reflex is negative; cold water is instilled into the ear canal and the patient's response observed over 1–2 minutes; this is repeated on the other side after 5 minutes
  - 'positive' if intact; the patient's eyes will show slow conjugate deviation towards the instilled side
  - 'negative' suggests brainstem involvement
  - if the unconscious state is factitious then caloric testing will show nystagmus with the fast phase away from the instilled ear

Breathing pattern

The patient is likely to be ventilated; nonetheless, the spontaneous breathing pattern is informative. Ataxic breathing is a variable amplitude and rate and suggests lower brainstem dysfunction. Sustained hyperventilation indicates a midbrain lesion. Cheyne–Stokes respiration describes cycles of crescendo–descendo breathing with periods of apnoea, and occurs with diencephalic lesions (**Figure 10.1**).

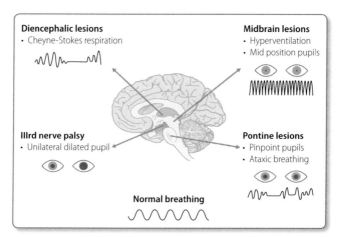

Figure 10.1 Pupil size and breathing pattern in comatose patients, depend of type of lesion. A unilateral pupil in a comatose patient suggests either a subarachnoid haemorrhage from an expanding posterior communicating artery aneurysm or raised intracranial pressure from any cause leading to transtentorial herniation.

Cortical lesions

Diffuse damage to either or both cerebral hemispheres from any cause can result in impaired consciousness. The key to identifying the lesion here is the posture and direction of gaze paresis.

Posture

Once admitted to hospital, the comatose patient has meticulous nursing care directed towards avoiding bedsores. This involves readjusting posture, so it is often difficult to interpret the 'natural' posture of the patient. The following may suggest the location of the lesion:

- **parietal lobe posture**: the patient neglects the affected side and may have their arm or leg in an awkward position
- **decorticate posture**: in a unilateral lesion the patient's:
  - contralateral arm is flexed
  - contralateral foot is slightly extended

- eyes are deviated away from the paresis and towards the hemispheric lesion
- in diffuse cortical dysfunction the signs above are bilateral with eyes in the midline (**Figure 10.2**)
- **brainstem hemiparetic posture**: in this the patient will have:
  - ipsilateral arm and/or leg paresis
  - eyes looking towards the lesion and paresis
- **decerebrate posture**: the patient's arms and legs are extended and internally rotated and this indicates a brainstem lesion (**Figure 10.3**)

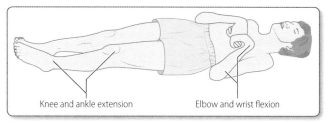

Knee and ankle extension   Elbow and wrist flexion

Figure 10.2 Decorticate posturing.

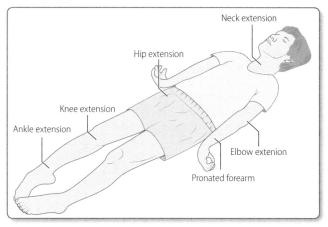

Neck extension

Hip extension

Knee extension

Ankle extension

Elbow extension

Pronated forearm

Figure 10.3 Decerebrate posturing.

10.4 General observations

Objective

General observations will help to:
- determine the patient's level of consciousness
- identify the posture of the patient
- establish the degree and range of physiological support
- give clues to the underlying cause

Approach

Assuming that the patient has been resuscitated and is stable, proceed to determine the Glasgow Coma Scale (GCS) score first to determine how co-operative the patient will be.

Equipment

This requires a stethoscope.

Sequence

Perform a targeted general examination:

1. in an examination situation ask the examiner whether the patient is otherwise stable and has had their cervical spine cleared
2. determine their GCS score (**Table 10.1**)
3. note any intravenous infusions, including sedatives
4. inspect the patient
   - **skin**: cyanosis, pallor, cherry redness, jaundice, petechiae, uraemic frost
   - **skull**: blood in the ear canal, Battle's sign, racoon eyes, cerebrospinal fluid (CSF)
   - **temperature**: pyrexia, hypothermia
   - **meningism**: resistance to passive neck flexion and extension
   - **breathing pattern**: note the ventilator settings, Cheyne–Stokes respiration, ataxic, hyperventilation
   - **posture**
5. general examination
   - pulse, blood pressure, heart sounds
   - respiratory rate, breath sounds, oxygen saturations

Component	Score
Eyes open	
Spontaneously	4
To verbal stimulation	3
To pain	2
Never	1
Best verbal response	
Orientated and converses	5
Disorientated and converses	4
Inappropriate words	3
Incomprehensive sounds	2
No response	1
Best motor response	
Obeys commands	6
Localises pain	5
Withdraws to pain	4
Flexes to pain	3
Extends to pain	2
No response	1
Total	15

Table 10.1 The Glasgow Coma Scale

Key differential diagnoses

Common causes of coma include:

- **raised intracranial pressure**
- **meningitis/encephalitis**: rash, fever, meningism
- **seizure**: sedation for status epilepticus, lateral tongue bitten, may have post-ictal hemiparesis, incontinence
- **poisoning**: there are a wide range of haemodynamic signs depending on the poison. Opiates may cause pin-point pupils, low respiratory rate and needle tracks
- **trauma**: there may be signs of: (1) head injury; (2) base of skull fracture – bruising around the eyes (racoon eyes) or behind the ears (Battle's sign), CSF leak from the ear or nose; and (3) fracture of long bones or ribs
- **metabolic**: there are a myriad of clinical signs, including: (1) uraemic frost in renal failure, jaundice and stigmata of liver

disease in hepatic encephalopathy; and (2) sepsis may progress to encephalopathy or require sedation and ventilation
- **stroke**: decorticate or decerebrate posture

What happens next?
Next, move on to examining the eyes and reflexes.

10.5 Eyes and reflexes

Objective
This examination determines whether the brainstem is affected or remains intact.

Approach
Ensure that the C-spine has been cleared of any injury by asking the examiner or checking X-rays or CT scans.

Equipment
This requires a pen torch, tendon hammer, cotton wool and a syringe with cold water.

Sequence
To examine the eyes and reflexes of a patient in a coma:
1. note any gaze paresis
2. note any spontaneous eye opening or eye movements
3. open the patient's eyelids if they are closed and observe
4. ask the patient to look up, down, left, right
5. oculocephalic reflexes: turn the patient's head to the right, left, up and down and observe whether their eyes move (**Figure 10.4**)
6. test the blink reflex
7. note the resting pupil sizes
8. elicit the pupillary reflexes
9. examine tone in the limbs
10. elicit triceps, biceps, knee, ankle and plantar reflexes
11. elicit oculovestibular reflexes (caloric reflexes) if the above fails to demonstrate an intact brainstem (**Figure 10.5**).

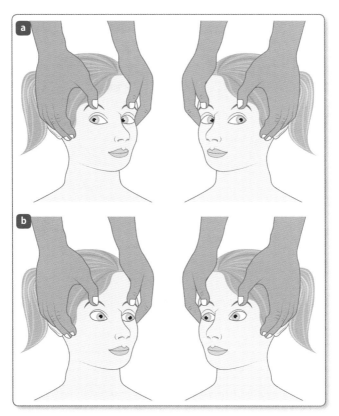

Figure 10.4 Oculocephalic reflexes. (a) As the head is turned one way the normal response is for the eyes to deviate in the opposite direction so as to maintain fixation at a given point. (b) Absence of this normal reflex results in the eyes turning with the head. This indicates brainstem dysfunction.

Key differential diagnoses
Gaze paresis and eye movements

Signs of eye deviation and movement can indicate the location of the lesion:

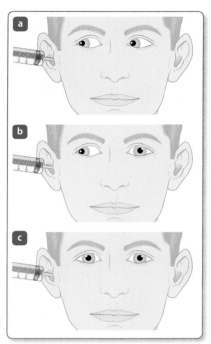

Figure 10.5
Oculovestibular reflexes
(a) When cold water is instilled into one ear the normal response is for the eyes to slowly deviate towards that side. (b) In lesions of the medial longitudinal fasciculus (MLF) in the brainstem, there is failure of the eye to abduct on the side ipsilateral to the instilled ear. (c) Failure of either eye to move indicates brainstem dysfunction.

- eyes deviated towards the hemiparetic side: the patient's eyes look towards the side of a brainstem lesion
- eyes deviated away from the hemiparetic side: the patient's eyes look away from the side of a cerebral hemisphere lesion
- eyes below the midline: this suggests a midbrain lesion
- skew deviation (one eye lower than the other): there is a medulla or pontine lesion ipsilateral to the down eye or basal ganglia or thalamic lesion contralateral to the down eye

- both eyes adducted: this indicates a bilateral VIth nerve palsy from raised intracranial pressure
- occular bobbing: this indicates a pontine lesion
- tracking: the patient will track movement in the horizontal plane if the midbrain is intact

Clinical insight

The locked-in syndrome occurs when the ventral pons is damaged but the anterior portion is spared. The descending corticospinal tracts are damaged and completely paralyse the patient but the reticular activating system is intact and the patient is conscious. There is variable sparing of ocular movements, typically with preserved upgaze or eyelid movements, meaning that the patient can communicate through blinking or eye movements.

Pupils

Pupil signs and their associated lesions are given above in section 10.3.

Tone and limb reflexes

A number of signs can indicate the location of the lesion:
- Normal: there is a diffuse toxic or metabolic cause
- cortical lesion: weakness is worse contralateral to the lesion. Reflexes are brisk. The patient may be acutely flaccid and then spastic
- cerebellar lesion: often quadriplegic. Reflexes are brisk. The patient may be acutely flaccid and then spastic

Oculovestibular reflexes (caloric reflexes)

These can indicate whether the brainstem is involved or not:
- intact reflex suggests that some basic function of the brainstem remains
- absent reflexes suggests that the brainstem is involved and carries a very poor prognosis

What happens next?

Direct investigations towards determining the underlying cause.

10.6 System summary

Examination of a patient in a coma is summarised in **Table 10.2**.

Inspection	Check C-spine
	Glasgow Coma Scale score
	Intravenous infusions and physiological support
	Patient: skin, skull, neck, mouth, temperature, breathing, posture
General examination	Cardiovascular
	Respiratory
Eyes and reflexes	Gaze paresis
	Eye movements
	Oculocephalic reflexes
	Blink reflex
	Pupillary reflexes
	Limb tone
	Limb reflexes
	Oculovestibular reflexes

Table 10.2 Examining a patient in a coma

The neurological screening examination in 4 minutes

11.1 Objectives

There is seldom a good reason not to perform a brief neurological examination on any patient admitted to hospital for any cause. Even in those without any neurological symptoms it is important to establish and document baseline gross neurological function and potentially detect any significant pathology.

In a busy outpatient setting, many consultant neurologists only need to perform a very brief screening examination. This is because they usually already know the diagnosis from the history (or so they would have you believe!) and are expert at interpreting any signs that are present.

The following is a simple ordered list of the important steps to include in such screening examinations. The detailed techniques are all covered in previous chapters. This may seem like a lot to do on every patient but, once well-rehearsed, such a screening can be done in 2–3 minutes.

11.2 Sequence

A summary of the sequence of performing a neurological screening examination is given in **Table 11.1**.

Handedness	'Are you left or right handed?'
Orientation	'What is the year? Month? Day? Date? Where are you?
Gait	Ask the patient to walk to the end of the room and back
Speech	Ask them to touch their left cheek with their right thumb
	Ask them to say 'baby', 'hippopotamus' and 'education'
Neck stiffness	Ask the patient to flex, extend and rotate their neck to assess for meningism
CN II–XII	Assess the patient's pupils
	Assess their fields
	Check their fundi for papilloedema
	Assess their range of eye movements
	Assess their sensation on the face and their strength of teeth clenching
	Check their facial movements: 'lift your eyebrows, close your eyes tight, show me your teeth'
	Look in their mouth and observe their palate
	Ask them to cough
Upper limb	Tone
	Power: deltoids, biceps, triceps, wrist extension, finger extension, finger abduction, finger flexion, opponens pollicis
	Reflexes: biceps, triceps, suppinator
	Co-ordination: finger–nose pointing
	Sensation: pin-prick and vibration
Lower limb	Tone
	Power: hip flexion, extension, adduction, abduction, knee flexion and extension, ankle dorsiflexion and plantarflexion
	Reflexes: knee, ankle, plantars
	Co-ordination: heel–shin
	Sensation: pin-prick and vibration

Table 11.1 A neurological screening examination

The neurological examination in undergraduate exams

12.1 Objectives

The aim of undergraduate clinical examinations is to ensure a basic standard of competency and to offer students an opportunity to demonstrate particular aptitude. Both of these will only be developed through practice: there is no substitute for rehearsing the examination routine on real patients. Examiners do not often expect nuanced skill or the ability to discuss the more subtle points of the neurological examination. Rather, they want to see students who have a clear grasp of a basic, but thorough, examination routine.

For those students with a keen interest in neurology or a wish to excel in the clinic examination, the key is to be sufficiently practised in the routines described here to be able to carry them out correctly and quickly in order to spend more time on questions with the examiners. Spending time attempting to elicit fine points of the examination is less impressive than finishing quickly, having a sensible summary and differential, and then being able to discuss investigations and management.

So the key to basic competency is practice, and the key to standing out is even more practice! In the immediate run-up to examinations it is often helpful to pair up and examine a fellow student repeatedly until the routine is slick, fast and second nature. Of course, without seeing real patients beforehand, any real signs found in the actual examination will prove more difficult to interpret.

12.2 Common conditions in examinations

The conditions which examiners like to offer students are those that are common, stable and with clear signs. You are unlikely to be offered the patient with meningitis, coma (although students have been known to be taken to ITU for their examination!) or subarachnoid haemorrhage. However, examiners are also known for their fondness for rare syndromes, so you may also see patients with neurofibromatosis, acromegaly (with bilateral carpel tunnel syndrome) or polymyositis.

Conditions commonly seen in examinations that students need to be very familiar with include:

- neurofibromatosis
- Friedreich's ataxia
- multiple sclerosis
- headache history
- stroke
- seizure history
- diabetic neuropathy
- myasthenia gravis
- Parkinson's disease
- Bell's palsy
- polymyositis

12.3 Examination instructions

Even a brief neurological screening examination can take up most of the time allowed in an examination setting, so examiners often ask for a very limited part of the examination to be performed, e.g. 'Please examine sensation in this patient's legs' or 'Please examine this patient's eyes'. This can be disarming for students who have rehearsed routines as a whole rather than as modular components, but this is common in examinations and is to be expected. If the instructions seem unclear, feel free to ask for clarification, e.g. 'Would you like me to examine all aspects of the eyes or just movement?'

12.4 Questions and answers

After presenting the findings, the student will be asked a series of questions. Typically, the examiners will start off with fairly basic questions about differential diagnosis, investigation and management. Answers should be brief and sensible: give common conditions first rather than obscure conditions. It is worth knowing two or three differential diagnoses for the presentations commonly encountered along with the initial investigations.

Examiners will ask increasingly difficult questions to find the limit of the student's knowledge. Since they usually know a lot more than the student being examined, this often ends with the student answering 'I don't know' to a question. The temptation is then to feel that one has done poorly in the examination; however, this is the inevitable endpoint and simply means the examiners were testing as far as they could go. Do not be discouraged!

A final point is to be aware of current recommendations from the relevant driving license authority (e.g. the Driver and Vehicle Licensing Agency in the UK) on conditions such as stroke/transient ischaemic attack and seizures as examiners often ask about these.

Further reading

Clinical neurology and neurosurgery

Brazis PW, Masdeu JC, Biller J. Localization in Clinical Neurology, 7th edn. Philadelphia: Lippincott Williams & Wilkins, 2016.

Brust J. Current Diagnosis and Treatment: Neurology, 2nd edition. New York: McGraw-Hill Education, 2011.

Collins D, Goodfellow J, Silva D, Dardis R, Nagaraja S. Eureka Neurology and Neurosurgery. London: JP Medical, 2016.

The Guarantors of Brain. Aids to Examination of the Peripheral Nervous System, 4th edn. Philadelphia: Saunders, 2000.

Neuroanatomy

Haines DE. Neuroanatomy in Clinical Context: An Atlas of Structures, Sections, Systems and Syndromes, 9th edition. Philadelphia: Lippincott Williams & Wilkins, 2014.

Hirsch M, Kramer T. Neuroanatomy: 3-D Stereoscopic Atlas of the Human Brain. Berlin: Springer, 1999.

Basic neuroscience

Cooper JR, Bloom FE, Roth RH. The Biochemical Basis of Neuropharmacology, 8th edn. New York: Oxford University Press, 2003.

Kandel E, Schwartz, JH, Jessell TM. Principles of Neural Science, 4th edn. New York: McGraw-Hill, 2000.

Shephard GM. The Synaptic Organization of the Brain, 5th edn. New York: Oxford University Press, 2004.

Psychiatry

Burton, N. Psychiatry, 3rd edn. Oxford: Wiley-Blackwell, 2016.

Folstein MF, Folstein SE, McHugh PR. 'Mini-mental state'. A practical method for grading the cognitive state of patients for the clinician. J Psychiatr Res 1975; 12:189–98.

Mind–brain philosophy

Eccles JC, Popper K. The Self and Its Brain. Abingdon, UK: Routledge, 2003.

Index

Note: Page numbers in **bold** or *italic* refer to tables or figures respectively.